David J. Ahearn, DDS

Dental Office Start-Up Guide

Your key to practice success

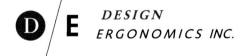

DESIGN
ERGONOMICS INC.

Design Ergonomics, Inc.
198 Airport Road, Fall River, MA 02720

800.275.2547
www.desergo.com

PRAISE FROM DENTAL OFFICE OWNERS

"Whether you are a new dentist, or on the cusp of retirement, **there is wisdom in this book for everyone.**"

Dr. Kate Raymond

Raymond Dental Group

"Congratulations for making it through dental school and beginning your journey in a rewarding career! But wait, what class was it in dental school that prepared you for practice ownership, training and managing staff, building an office, and scaling up a dental business? **If you embrace the principles of the design and workflow [in this book], you WILL be able to more quickly and fully achieve your business potential.**"

Dr. Jonah Barasz

Dental Implants & Periodontics of Connecticut

"We have seen a gross increase in production of 40% after our first full year in our new office. **The return of our investment has been overwhelming to the point of needing to develop more clinical space after only a year and hire more staff to keep up with growth.**"

Dr. Dallin Kay

Red Rock Dental

"Having been in our newest facility for 4 years now **we are still in love with our facility and with our inevitable expansion due to the success.**"

Dr. Ray Becker

Howard County Smiles

"All of the research and development Dr. Ahearn has curated over many years was turned into a book for someone just like me. I fully bought into their office plan, design, ergonomics - you name it. This made my search for real estate much more exciting and **gave me confidence that taking on a renovation/new office build was going to complete my vision by utilizing the ideas in the book.**"

Dr. Ty Milner

Milner Dentistry

CONTENTS

I wrote this book with clear memory of all of the joy and fear and determination that I had three decades ago prior to my own startup.

Back then, I really didn't have a choice. I was, apparently, not great associate material! Honestly, I would have loved to have been an associate - of mine anyway - Apparently that was not a possibility for me!

Today, emerging practitioners have many choices:

- Quality full and part time associateships in successful larger practices
- You can buy, rehabilitate and grow a fixer upper practice
- You can go corporate and punch the clock and have minimal responsibilities
- You can become a franchisee
- And you can also create your very own startup

This book is for the lucky few who every year recognize an opportunity to create your own vision. The dream practice that will launch your career, not just as a clinician but additionally, as a dental entrepreneur. This book contains all the lessons I wish I had known when I started out, plus many more that I've learned along the way, As the nation's largest independent dental office design firm each and every year we are fortunate enough to work with dozens of great doctors like yourself in creating these dreams. I am confident that with the writing of this book, with my long term coworker and collaborator Tim Gagnon, that your future can exceed your wildest expectations.

Here's to your greatest success!

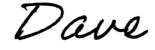

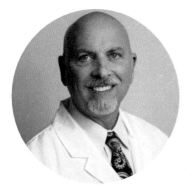

David J. Ahearn, DDS

1 THE DREAM PRACTICE

What's your dream as a dentist? What does your ideal dental practice look like?

From your first day in dental school, you probably had a picture in your mind. What kind of patients did you imagine treating? Kids? Entire families? Young adults? Wealthy older population? Or did you picture yourself as a general dentist or a specialist?

Your answers shape the look, feel, and even location of your practice. Let's say you're into General Family Dentistry. Being close to a school or a mall might be a smart move since that's where families hang out. If you're aiming to help young professionals, think about a spot in the city, close to offices, shops, and easy transportation.

But having a vision goes deeper. In the top-notch practices, everyone from the receptionist to the dentist can quickly tell you what the place stands for. Try this: walk into ten dental offices nearby and ask any team member, "What's the primary purpose here?" Chances are, you'll get some puzzled faces. Maybe a few will remember something their boss once mentioned. But it's rare to hear a clear, straight answer.

The cool part? This is totally in your hands. Sketch out your dream. Come up with a phrase or a couple of sentences that capture what you expect from yourself, your team, and your patients. Here's the thing – you're going to make a good living. All our clients do. But aim for more than just profit. Build a place you'd be proud to be part of, something that feels right for years to come.

From this main idea, you can branch out to other big concepts like Core Values or maybe a Mission Statement. A tip? Work on this with your team – it's a group thing. Write down your ideas and make them visible in the office. Seeing reminders of your vision and values helps keep everyone on the same page.

There's more to chat about, like how to keep your team inspired. We'll dive into that in the "Hiring & Training" section. But for now, think about these questions and see if your dream practice starts taking shape.

MAPPING OUT YOUR DREAM PRACTICE

1. **Your Dental Specialty**
   What kind of dental procedures make you excited?

2. **Your Ideal Patient**
   Who do you picture when you think about the perfect patient? Kids with their first tooth? Athletes needing protection? Retirees looking for a brighter smile? The working professional needing restorative work? For more information, refer to our chapter on Site Selection and Demographics.

3. **Team Values**
   Think about qualities that really matter to you. What traits do you hope to see in the people

working beside you every day? Honesty? Openness? Punctuality? Write them down and show them to potential hires. You will learn more about values in our chapter on Hiring, Training, & Retention.

4. Community Image

Picture someone nearby chatting about your clinic. What's the first thing you hope they would say?

5. Your Favorite Procedures

Are there certain procedures you're especially passionate about? And on the flip side, are there any you'd rather avoid?

6. Why Join Your Team?

If someone is considering working at your practice, what's the big draw? Why is your place special?

7. Choosing You

Picture a potential patient weighing their options. Why should they pick you as their dentist?

Once you've mulled over these questions, take a quiet moment. Let everything sink in and ask yourself, "What's my vision for my practice?" See if a clear picture or theme jumps out at you.

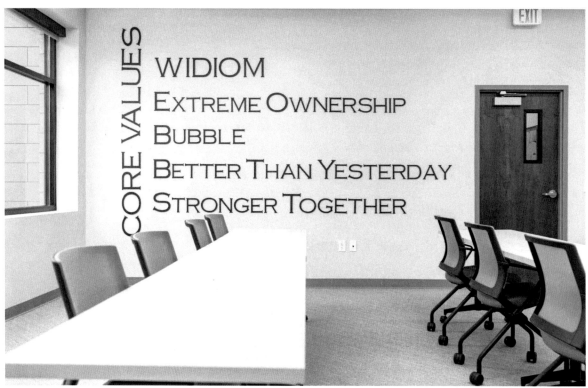

Private dental practice provides incredible opportunities to turn a vision into reality.

2 WHY BUILD A DENTAL PRACTICE?

Although individual reasons for starting a dental practice may differ from one dentist to another, there's a universal set of benefits that come with taking this step. Here are some of the standout advantages:

OWNERSHIP

Ever felt that certain decisions made in your workplace were not in line with your professional or personal values? This might relate to clinical choices, team management, patient care, or business practices. Owning your own practice gives you full control over all these decisions. It's a kind of freedom mainly available to small business owners and can pave the way to true self-fulfillment. However, a word of caution: before diving in, consider reading Michael Gerber's "The E Myth Revisited: Why Most Small Businesses Don't Work and What to Do About It." Many believe they can avoid the pitfalls of their previous employers, only to encounter the same issues they thought they were leaving behind.

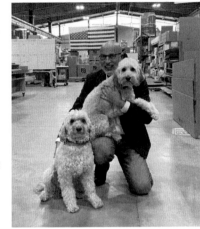

Dr. David J. Ahearn, DDS at Design Ergonomics in Fall River, MA.

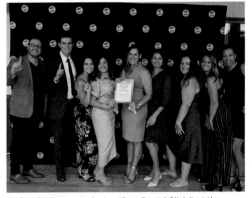

Perfect Smiles team winning "Best Dental Clinic" at the SouthCoast Community's Choice Awards.

GROWING OTHERS

As a business owner, you have the privilege of assembling, mentoring, and nurturing a team. Although the process might have its challenges, over time, it's incredibly rewarding to witness the growth of individuals. Over the span of 5, 10, or even 20 years, you can see young team members evolve into responsible adults, starting families and building legacies. You might have employees who are the first in their family to finish college, purchase a home, or travel abroad. Through your mentorship and support, you're not just running a business, you're shaping lives.

REAL ESTATE AND TAX ADVANTAGES

While this isn't the main focus, running a business brings numerous financial benefits. These include building equity, enjoying tax deductions & credits, transforming personal expenses into business costs, appreciating and depreciating assets, and accessing better credit terms. As your business matures, you'll also find that you can secure more favorable terms from vendors and creditors. All these benefits position

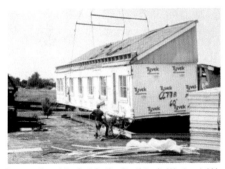

Construction at Perfect Smiles Dentistry in Westport, MA was completed in 30 days.

you well for future investments or acquisitions. To maximize these advantages, it's often advisable to own the property your business operates from. While this might not be feasible for many startups (kudos if it's possible for you!), it's a goal that many dentists should aim for within a 5-to-10-year time frame.

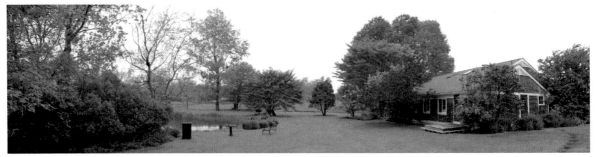

Perfect Smiles Dentistry in Westport, MA was Dr. Ahearns original startup.

COMMUNITY ENGAGEMENT

Providing quality and compassionate oral health care to the residents of your city or town is a noble goal. In a country where private practitioners face increasing pressures, the success of the vast majority (95% to be precise) showcases a more patient-centric approach to dentistry. Such practices, prioritizing individuals over profits, often become trusted and respected institutions in their communities for many years.

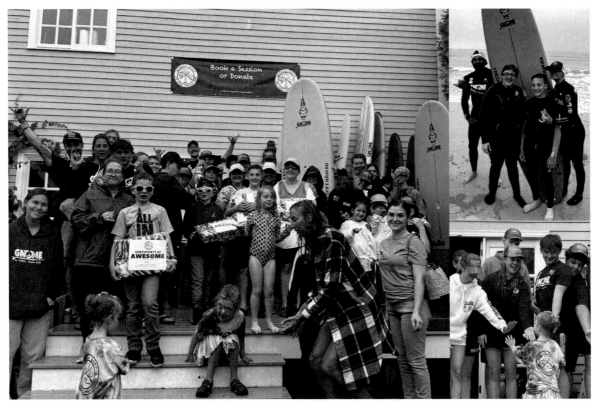

Perfect Smiles at Gnome Surf Happy Camp - A 501c3 Nonprofit Surf Therapy Organization for all abilities.

POTENTIAL FOR INCREASED INCOME

As an associate, you probably earn roughly 30% of your adjusted production. After accounting for overhead costs, which range from 40%-50%, the practice likely nets a profit margin of 10%-20%. As the owner of a practice, this net income would be yours. The ADA's most recent data reveals that the average Solo GP earns $160k annually, while the average employed dentist brings in $126k. This difference in earnings is what you can aim to bridge by venturing into ownership. It's worth noting that many earn significantly more than the average figures. In fact, if you choose to work with us, we expect and hope to see you at least double that income in a relatively short time.

THE THREE PILLARS OF SUCCESS

Over the past 30 years, we've worked with numerous doctors at various stages in their careers. They've sought our assistance with the design, equipment selection, and system development for their dental practices. This could be for a renovation, an expansion, a brand-new start-up, or any additional practice they wish to add to their portfolio. Interestingly, some doctors manage to realize their vision and complete their project more effortlessly than others. What makes the difference? Although numerous factors contribute to a successful outcome—like having a competent team, setting a realistic timeframe, demonstrating resilience and flexibility, and utilizing systems and checklists—we've noticed that three factors distinctly stand out. By ensuring you're strong in these three pivotal areas, you'll be setting yourself on the path to a successful dental office project.

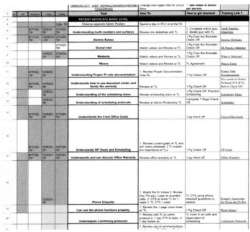

It is important to utilize systems and checklists to ensure consistency and efficiency in your practice.

1. FINANCIAL HEALTH

The reality is straightforward: if you're financially unstable, securing a loan to initiate your practice becomes challenging. Here's a general roadmap that most financial experts recommend:

A. Emergency Fund - Both Business and Personal

Aim to have liquid assets covering six months of expenses. To calculate this, multiply your monthly expenses by six and deposit that amount in an easily accessible account. Ensure you maintain an accurate personal budget. If you've yet to establish a monthly budget, you can start by downloading our budget template from the Resources section. Ideally, before embarking on this journey, you should have at least $50k in liquid assets and minimal personal debts, such as those from credit cards, car loans, and other personal loans or your primary residence mortgage.

B. Debt Management

Strive to reduce or completely eliminate personal debts, such as those from credit cards or car loans. However, don't be overly concerned about professional debts like student loans.

C. Determining Cash Flow

With your budget in place, ascertain your current cash flow. To do this, subtract your monthly expenses from your post-tax gross income. This will give you a clear picture of your net cash flow.

D. Increasing Cash Flow

This can be achieved by either increasing your income, reducing expenses, or both.

What's an ideal cash flow indicating you're prepared for a construction project? While this can fluctuate based on location, you should ideally have at least $2k/month surplus after covering all expenses. A surplus of $4k/month is even better. For instance, if you're an average ADA dentist with an annual net income of $160k, your yearly expenses should ideally not exceed $80k or $6,500 monthly.

When all your non-investment related expenses are settled each month, and you've successfully saved six months' worth of expenses for emergencies, any surplus, ideally at least $2k monthly, should be directed into your "investment" fund. This fund plays a critical role—it's what we'll tap into to finance the office project. Store this money in a low-risk liquid account. At the time of writing this, 3-month T-Bills are hovering around 5%, that would be a good option for this placement. Money Market or traditional savings accounts are also fine, but with slightly better access and lower returns.

Why the emphasis on $2k monthly? We use this benchmark because it approximates half of the overall loan payment the business would need to cover for the project. The goal is to ensure that you, as a dedicated working dentist, can comfortably manage at least half of this cost at your current production rate. And yes, we do anticipate boosting that rate over time.

As your business matures, first-time patients become loyal referrers. Your clinical team synchronizes, and appointments get booked well in advance. At this stage, it's wise to transfer the remaining mortgage responsibility solely to the business. After 3-5 years, consider refinancing—a move that offers various benefits. You could opt for a cash-out refinance, continue working with a lucrative 30%+ take-home rate, shift towards an associate-driven model with around 10% take-home, plan for business expansion or even strategize for a future sale or succession.

However, embarking on this venture isn't for everyone. If you're grappling with substantial personal debt, if your cash flow is barely noticeable, or if you're stretching your work hours just to stay afloat, then constructing an office might not be for you. Yet, financial strains can negatively impact the project. You might prioritize cheap options over experienced ones, be swayed by sales or discounts instead of dependable systems, or choose DIY routes over expert solutions. This can lead to ballooning costs in the long term due to lost revenue and subpar production. All this might land you in a position where you're earning roughly the same you did before, but with added stress, risk, and liabilities.

If this last paragraph resonates with you, perhaps consider a more rewarding associateship. The dental industry is teeming with flourishing practices in search of dedicated and trustworthy associates—many of whom are our esteemed clients.

2. CLINICAL & MANAGERIAL EXPERTISE

Your current associateship might have provided varying levels of training when it comes to diagnosing, creating treatment plans, and effectively presenting cases. However, it's worth noting that many associates with just 1-2 years of experience may fall short in one or more of these areas.

Case Presentation

Patients will exhibit diverse responses, ranging from complete acceptance to outright resistance to treatment suggestions. Despite these varied reactions, it's vital to maintain a consistent approach: diagnose the whole mouth, formulate a comprehensive treatment plan, and present the entire proposal—with phases and alternatives—in an efficient manner. Ultimately, while some patients might opt for the most basic solution, a consistent approach will yield more affirmative responses. This not only boosts your confidence and bottom line but also lays down a standardized system for future practitioners to emulate. Remember, you have the flexibility to refer out specific procedures that you're not keen on handling personally.

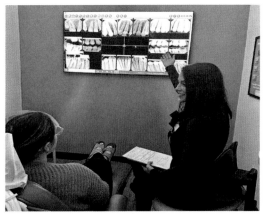

Chairside consultation is often the most comfortable way for the patient to understand and accept treatment.

Getting Your Team Started

On the managerial side, there's a noticeable gap in the skill set of many startups, particularly concerning hiring, training, and nurturing staff members. In fact, many new business owners unintentionally stifle their initial growth by not hiring an adequate number of hygienists or not investing time in training their assistants. Thinking, "I'll handle the cleanings myself for the initial months," as a feasible strategy. However, once your schedule starts filling up, it's crucial to onboard a hygienist. Why settle for $130/ hr when you can potentially generate $1,000/ HR+? Given that a cleaning and placing a crown both consume roughly the same time, it's more lucrative to identify opportunities for more extensive treatments during hygiene appointments. Strategize to meet the demand of running two hygiene columns with seven patients

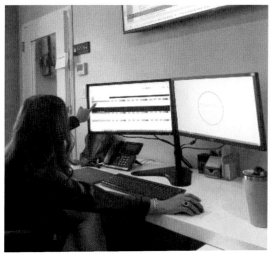

The team at your front desk should serve a Maître d' function rather than answering phones. Consider moving phones to a separate administrative areas.

each. This approach triples your diagnostic opportunities, potentially filling your calendar for days to come. A productive day of diagnosis can generate 2-3 days of restoration work.

Training

Another pivotal area that demands your attention is administrative training, especially for the front desk. Navigating the complexities of billing, coding, and insurance is paramount for seamless operations. Yet, remember, you pursued dental school for dentistry, not administration. Your aim should be to identify what stellar administration looks like—even if discerning this isn't your forte. Numerous competent administrators are eager to support a young, driven, expanding practice where their skills are acknowledged and rewarded.

Don't hesitate to discuss this domain with us. Our Over The Shoulder events provide our attendees with the opportunity to learn the techniques for increasing your productivity and show you the office and equipment design elements that make this possible. Investing in this guidance will prove invaluable.

3. AVOIDING BAD ADVICE

One of the big hurdles we see dentists face when starting their own practice is following the wrong advice. There are loads of salespeople, financial folks, real estate experts, and business advisors ready to help. With so many voices, it's tough to know who to listen to. Part of the reason we made this guide is because we saw too many doctors getting lost with bad advice. If you need advice on who to partner with, contact us. We collaborate closely with the best dealers and consultants in the dental industry.

When setting up your new office, there's a lot to think about. But let's focus on the must-haves. You'll need a:

- **Solid business plan**
- **Up-to-date financial statements**
- **Clear building plans**
- **The right equipment**

- **Detailed construction estimates**
- **A team to help you start**
- **The basic supplies**
- **The latest tech tools**

If you're working with a consultant or advisor, make sure they're really helping in these areas and not just talking. Just getting advice won't actually get your office up and running. We put this guide together to give you a lot of this info up front, without a big price tag. We believe good advice shouldn't be locked behind a paywall or the exclusive offering of some "guru." If you find this guide helpful, we think you'll also like what else we can offer in terms of services and solutions.

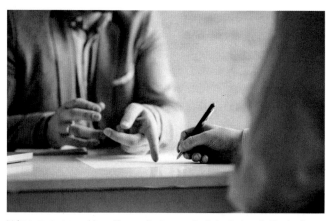

Make sure you are working with consultants you actually trust when starting to discuss building your own practice.

3 BUILDING THE TEAM

To successfully launch your startup, you'll need the expertise of various specialized individuals. Each contributes a unique and vital part of the overall workload. It's essential to see these as potential long-term professional relationships that might last for many years. Investing time early on to choose people you trust and enjoy working with can significantly benefit your dental practice's success and growth.

Before diving deeper, we should heed some crucial advice about building the team. While there are many elements to consider, one of the surest ways to hinder success is by having too many decision-makers. A proficient Design Build firm can serve as the architect, contractor, and project manager simultaneously. This not only helps in cost reduction but, more critically, shortens the time to completion.

ATTORNEY

Your attorney plays a crucial role in ensuring all your legal bases are covered. They will review pivotal documents like the lease, articles of incorporation, employee contracts, and service agreements. Moreover, if any disputes or litigations arise during the construction process, your attorney will be instrumental (though with proper planning, such situations should be rare). Start with a real estate or business attorney, as their expertise will be more relevant than, say, a family law or accident specialist. Be cautious: if your new attorney starts suggesting more consultants, remember you're still building trust and aren't best friends yet!

ACCOUNTANT

A CPA with experience in the dental field can be a game-changer. They will prepare personal financial statements for lenders, draft company financial statements like Profit & Loss and Balance Sheets, assist in establishing your business entity, file for incorporation, prepare tax returns, and regularly review financial activity. However, be careful! While accountants provide essential financial expertise, they almost never have an entrepreneurial mindset. They might sometimes encourage you to think smaller or more conservatively than your vision dictates.

REALTOR/LEASE NEGOTIATOR

As you search for the perfect location for your practice, consider enlisting the services of a commercial realtor or lease negotiator. They can pinpoint available spaces matching your criteria and commence negotiations with potential landlords. If you're struggling to find one, feel free to contact us; we likely have resources to recommend.

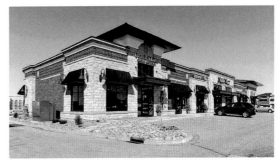

The right strip center has potential for exposure and traffic flow.

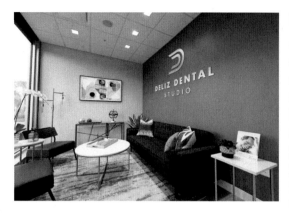

DENTAL OFFICE DESIGNER

Once you've zeroed in on a space, a designer's expertise becomes invaluable. They can quickly conduct "test fits" of the space to ensure it accommodates your requirements. Preliminary layouts can be drawn up to confirm the area's suitability. A top-notch designer will remain by your side throughout the project, serving as your advocate when dealing with other involved parties. And, just so you know, we pride ourselves on being unparalleled in this domain.

ARCHITECT

The requirement of an architect may vary by municipality and sometimes the landlord/contractor is able to control the permitting process. None-the-less we often find that coordination of approvals and perhaps code compliance can be best handled by a local, licensed professional.

GENERAL CONTRACTOR/DESIGN BUILD FIRM

Your general contractor bears the responsibility of physically bringing your dental office vision to life. They hire suitable subcontractors and tradesmen, provide you with the total construction cost, and collaborate with the designer and architect to ensure timely completion within the budget. Engaging a contractor familiar with dental office requirements is advisable. If, however, they've mainly built "Room Centric" practices, their estimates will be higher based on their experience with such projects. (The difference between "Room vs. Office centric" will be detailed in chapter 6 - Office Design.) We may be able to recommend a seasoned Design/Build professional in your vicinity.

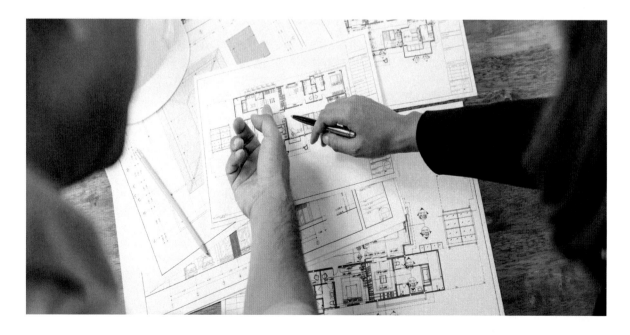

DENTAL EQUIPMENT REPRESENTATIVE

This role revolves around sourcing the specialized equipment and technology tailored for dental practices. Your representative communicates with one or more dental equipment vendors, helping you equip your treatment rooms, sterilization areas, labs, mechanical rooms, and fulfill your tech needs. Choose vendors based on their capacity to meet your performance and productivity aspirations. Be cautious: it's not the job of dental "salespeople" to dictate the equipment essentials for your new practice. Your budgeting for this segment requires keen attention and strategic planning.

SUPPLY COMPANY

Analogous to the equipment reps, you'll collaborate with one or more dental supply firms. They will furnish the sundry supplies, materials, disposables, instruments, burrs, and so forth for your new adventure. We advocate for well-established, direct- to - consumer companies known for competitive prices and swift delivery times. For a comprehensive list of anticipated supplies for your startup, refer to the supplies & inventory section.

IT SPECIALIST

Often an external consultant, the IT person will collaborate with the General Contractor to set up all technological systems pivotal to your practice. Their purview encompass phone systems, computer workstations, servers, software (including practice management software), and possibly digital imaging systems. They might also oversee the setup of sound and security systems. In our tech-driven age, their role is indispensable for a smoothly running dental practice.

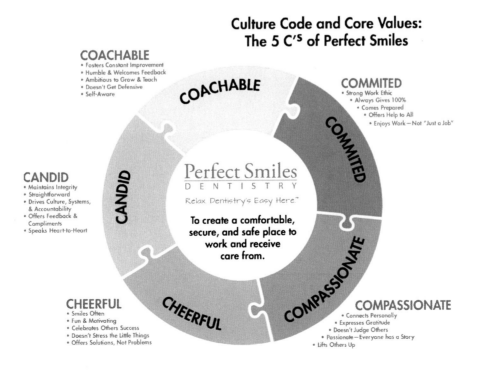

**Culture Code and Core Values:
The 5 C's of Perfect Smiles**

COACHABLE
- Fosters Constant Improvement
- Humble & Welcomes Feedback
- Ambitious to Grow & Teach
- Doesn't Get Defensive
- Self-Aware

COMMITED
- Strong Work Ethic
- Always Gives 100%
- Comes Prepared
- Offers Help to All
- Enjoys Work — Not "Just a Job"

CANDID
- Maintains Integrity
- Straightforward
- Drives Culture, Systems, & Accountability
- Offers Feedback & Compliments
- Speaks Heart-to-Heart

Perfect Smiles
D E N T I S T R Y
Relax Dentistry's Easy Here.™

To create a comfortable, secure, and safe place to work and receive care from.

CHEERFUL
- Smiles Often
- Fun & Motivating
- Celebrates Others Success
- Doesn't Stress the Little Things
- Offers Solutions, Not Problems

COMPASSIONATE
- Connects Personally
- Expresses Gratitude
- Doesn't Judge Others
- Passionate — Everyone has a Story
- Lifts Others Up

4 HOW TO HIRE A CONTRACTOR

The third potential hurdle, after planning/vision and financials, we see dentists face when embarking on building or renovating a dental practice is the necessary step of finding, vetting and hiring a General Contractor (GC) to perform the physical construction. In this article we'll outline some of the more important considerations and steps you should take when embarking on this phase of your Dental Office project.

Before we begin with the criteria and characteristics required of a good GC let's first explain what a GC does, why we need one and why we can't just round up our college buddies, get a few cases of beer and 100 trips to Home Depot later have a Dental Office up and running.

WHAT IS A GENERAL CONTRACTOR?

A GC is a professional title held by individuals (or business entities) in the construction industry responsible for overseeing a construction project. Like practicing dentistry, most states require that contractors engaging in significant construction projects (those requiring building permits) be Licensed and Insured. To obtain these licenses these professionals often need to pass a state issued examination, have a few thousand hours or relevant training & experience and remain in good standing with their regulatory body. Including completing required continuing education as well as maintaining adequate insurance.

In states without specific GC licensing requirements (Vermont for example) individual municipalities can legislate the need for licenses at the trade level such as for electrical and plumbing work. Even in these cases there will still be a GC who is responsible for hiring these subcontractors and coordinating the overall project.

Procore – a valuable construction management software – has a comprehensive list of contractor requirements by state. Check this first to see what's necessary in your state.

WHAT DOES A GC DO?

There's an awful lot that goes into this but in short, they build the building and perform all the necessary tasks around building the building, including but not limited to;

- Engages with the client and designers regarding design considerations
- Performs various surveys and measurements of the current conditions
- Verifies build-ability and feasibility of projects
- Provides the owner and lender with construction costs and estimates
- Hires and coordinates all subcontractors and tradesmen needed
- Purchases all materials, equipment and machinery
- Pulls building permits and schedules pertinent inspections
- Is obligated to perform all said work within the context and framework of the contract

WHY DO I NEED A GC?

In most states and municipalities, you're legally required to use a GC to build anything, whether it's a dental office or a bike shed. If it requires building permits, it usually requires a contractor. Now it's not the purpose of this article to debate what types of projects should and should not require building permits, but just know that almost ANY amount of construction inside of a commercial building, legally, requires permits. From adding light fixtures to moving a wall, literally anything that "constructs, reconstructs, alters, repairs, removes or demolishes a building, structure or portion thereof" will require a building permit.

Please note that attempting to avoid or circumvent this requirement is a crime in most jurisdictions punishable by fines and/or imprisonment, as well as possibly having to demolish any work done not under a permit and being forced to start over. Not to mention that if anything ever goes wrong during construction, if proper permits and licenses are not available, insurance companies will absolutely deny responsibility and leave the owner 100% liable for rectifying the matter.

HOW TO FIND A GC?

Before we hire them, first we have to find them, and there's a few different methods that have proven successful in the past to find potential contractors to build your next office we'll just list a few of the more common ones:

Ask Your Colleagues

Odds are, you're not the only dentist in your area to build a dental office, every other office at some point, had to hire a contractor to build or renovate their current spaces. Check with any friends, mentors, fellowship, or any other dentist in your area that might have a recommendation. If you can't find anyone in your circle that knows of someone you can try popular web forums like those on Dental Town, which has it's own Office Design & Construction section or Facebook Groups like Nifty Thrifty Dentists or Making of a Dental Startup to see if there's anyone in your state that might have a recommendation.

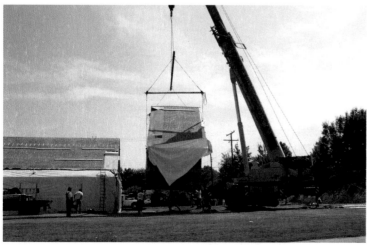

Modular construction is one of the techniques to accelerate project completion.

Google Search

Since the turn of the millennium, the internet of course is the best source for information we currently have at our disposal. Likewise, companies that realize this, have spent significant time and money on establishing a "web presence" to help potential prospects find them. While simply typing "General contractor in my area" will yield a list of candidates, digging further into a few specific areas will help separate the wheat from the chafe.

Website

How does their website look? Is it modern? Fresh? Loads quickly? Does it have a good portfolio section? Does it have FAQ's or Meet the Team sections? Or does it look like it was made 25 years ago on a free web builder? There's no reason a well-established successful contractor can't have a halfway decent website, be leery of those that don't.

Unsolicited Reviews. As in, the ones NOT on their own website. If they've done more than a handful of projects, odds are people have started leaving Google Reviews. Check them out and see what other people are saying, are they good, bad? Does the company itself respond when warranted?

Social Media

While not as indicative to performance as a good website, it's helpful to check their social media presence, if any. A simple, clean Facebook page with relevant posts, or a LinkedIn page listing their accolades or maybe they even have a YouTube channel where they post videos of projects are all signs of a company that cares about their reputation and delivering value to the potential customer. Consider this a "nice-to-have".

In Network Referrals

This one is the toughest to advocate for as it's the category we, Design Ergonomics would fall under, but it can also be one of the more dubious sources of contractor referral. In every community, synergistic businesses will keep a short (or long) list of referrals of people they would recommend to their clients for various needs. Realtors are notorious for this, need a plumber? Ask your Realtor. Someone to paint a bedroom? Realtor. A daycare to put the kids in so you can make your closing appointment, if your Realtor doesn't have one, they'll find one!

Likewise, even in the niche segment of construction that deals with Dental Offices, most established organizations will have a recommendation for another party member. Your supply rep might know a contractor, who knows an architect, who knows a financier, who knows an IT guy, who knows a cabinet guy, who knows a guy, etc. etc.

Sometimes, these various partners will have "backdoor" referral agreements with each other where they will pay, incentivize, spiff, bribe, whatever you want to call it, the originating source of the referral. In other words, they may be making recommendations based on personal motives as opposed to exclusively focusing on what's best for you the client.

This can be a difficult scenario to sniff out and get to the bottom of, but just know that anyone WITHOUT a financial reason for doing so, won't have a particularly strong opinion on who you use. Their recommendation should always come as more of a suggestion and never a mandate or obligation.

We at Design Ergonomics DON'T DO THIS! We have no financial arrangements or agreements with any of our construction industry partners or recommendations. At most we get a nice chocolate gift basket at Christmas time, (which we very much appreciate, please do not stop sending the chocolate!) What we do instead is, we only recommend people that we have had at least one successful project with. Since we work all across the US and Canada, we won't always have someone that meets this criteria in every municipality. If not, we are still happy to help vet potential candidates for our clients and we always review bids and construction estimates for free when asked.

HOW TO VET A GC?

Look up their license # and check the BBB. Most states with the requirement of licensure for contractors will have a contractor registration online portal where you can enter a contractor's license # and see if there are any past issues, suspensions or administrative actions. Additionally the Better Business Bureau performs a similar public service using the company name. Please note that individuals looking to bury past performance issues can always recreate their business entity or get a new license # under a new individual and sidestep this query. Be wary of businesses/individuals who have little to no history of business activities in your given area.

Ask for references and actually call them. Most contractors will be happy to provide a list of previous clients who can share their experiences with you. Do however ask for references that are relatively similar to the project you're undertaking, another dentist would be ideal but definitely former commercial clients, those who have developed similar sized projects would be beneficial. There's little to no value however in talking to someone who used them to build an expansion on their house or remodel their kitchen.

Go visit and look at their previous work. Calling folks and looking at portfolio images is great, but nothing beats seeing it in person. We learned this long ago in our Dental Office Designs and is one of the main reasons we offer Spotlight Clients instead of Showrooms, so you can actually see it in action, 100 or 1,000 days removed from Grand Opening. How is the construction methods holding up to the test of time? How does the front desk look? Lighting fixtures? Doors and windows? How's the HVAC system? Any plumbing or electrical issues? Don't worry so much about high traffic wear and tear items like flooring, furniture and countertops, those do and will get beat up over time but the bones of the building should still be in good condition 5, 10, or even 20 years later.

Evaluate their bidding process. Ask them how they bid on projects, what information do they need and to what level of accuracy do they offer on various levels of bids. We know that a bid on a floor plan might differ from the final construction estimate based off a 30 page permit plan set but why and how will they differ.

(HINT: material selections, mechanical systems, plumbing and lighting fixture selections, etc. will all help nail down a construction estimate but these items likely won't be known when you're just trying to get an idea of costs for a potential project) Do they have a formula? Can they share it? What sort of allowances are they providing for which areas? How are these allowances determined?

Have an attorney review the contract. We've seen some interesting construction contracts in our 25+ years of experience. From 1 pagers that say little more than "Dental office for $2M Sign here." to 20+ page legal dissertations. Contractors typically write contracts to protect themselves, just like you should never sign the first draft of a lease provided by a landlord, you shouldn't sign the first contract provided by a contractor. Have an attorney review it, have us review it and make sure that you are also protected in the areas that are most important to you, usually the areas involving money. How are they paid, how is performance calculated, how are change orders or price overages handled, , what happens if they finish early, what happens if they run over time, how are disputes settled, etc. Unfortunately a good contract (or should I say a bad one) can be worth millions of dollars in the end and it's imperative that this critical step be scrutinized by people whom you've retained to protect your interests.

Assess their subcontractor relationships. What subs do they use? Do they use the same subs on every job? Do they have a small pool from which they draw from? Do they sit outside Home Depot looking for trades people? And do said subs have experience with dental? You can hire the best GC in the world but if the plumbing sub doing your in slab work got his license yesterday, he might not know why it's important the vacuum line not have any 90 degree bends in it. It's worth asking who they use, why they use them and what kind of supervision will be in place.

P.S. Every GC, in the contract, should have a description of project supervision. Who is ultimately the person on the ground, who will be at the job site every day, representing the GC and coordinating the work to be performed. These folks typically hold titles of Foreman, Construction Manager, Project Manager, Site Supervisor, etc. and will be direct employees of the GC if not the GC themselves. Know who this person is as they will most likely be your #1 point of contact throughout the process. This person needs to be level-headed, accommodating and reachable. Make sure you know who this person will be prior to signing any contracts.

QUESTIONS TO ASK WHEN INTERVIEWING GC CANDIDATES
- How will project be staffed? List them and their roles.
- How will funds be dispersed? (no advance payments or forward funding)
- What is the meeting schedule and cadence? (bi-weekly, monthly, bi-monthly)
- How is progress measured and reported? (Procore, Gant Chart, etc.)

HOW TO REVIEW AN ESTIMATE AND CONTRACT
- Ensure all questions above have been answered adequately and are represented in the contract where applicable.
- Bid Project or Negotiated?

CAUSES & STIPULATIONS TO WATCH FOR
- Owned Retainment of Rights
- Architectural Drawings Referenced
- Lien waivers on major materials
- Lender dispersal process

WHAT TO AVOID WHEN HIRING A GC AND BUILDING A DENTAL OFFICE
- Don't hire a contractor outside your market area
- Don't hire a contractor with little or no dental/medical experience
- Don't avoid the construction site
- Don't pay for anything yourself

5 FINANCIALS & FINANCING

Before diving into the world of building a dental office, it's imperative to assess your financial health. Predominantly, lending institutions have specific creditworthiness criteria which determine not only if you qualify for a loan but also the loan amount.

LENDER REQUIREMENTS

1. **Experience as an Associate**
   Ideally, you should have at least two years of experience working as an associate, though one year can be accepted. For specialists, completing residency can be equivalent to associate experience. In fact, specialists might even secure financing immediately post-residency.

2. **Income Bracket**
   You should be on track to earn a minimum of $140,000 annually.

3. **Credit Card Debt**
   It's preferable to have zero personal credit card debt, though lenders typically accept up to $25,000.

4. **Student Loans**
   General dentists should have under $400,000 in outstanding student loans. For specialists, this figure rises to $500,000.

5. **Liquid Assets**
   Lenders expect you to have at least $40,000 in NET liquid assets, excluding debts. This sum should be present in bank accounts or in easily tradeable stocks and bonds. Funds in 401k and IRA accounts aren't counted. As a rule of thumb, the longer you've been practicing, the higher this liquid asset number should be. An increase of around $10,000 for each additional year is a reasonable estimate.

6. **Credit Application**
   Consult a Sample Credit Application to understand the specifics of the information you'll need to provide.

Currently, the ceiling loan amount for a startup practice from major lenders (e.g. Panacea) hovers around $700,000. This loan is typically divided into three primary expenses: construction, dental equipment & supplies, and working capital to cover six months.

It's worth noting that initial costs for designs and architectural plans aren't always enveloped within the standard startup loan. Confirm this with your lender, and be ready to consider a bridge loan if these costs aren't covered. Preliminary design and architectural plans could set you back anywhere from $20,000 to $40,000. And it's often challenging to procure comprehensive construction bids without these vital documents. As a strategic first step, we recommend getting a basic blocking diagram as a 'test fit' before you invest further in this segment.

Enlisting a reputable design-build firm can be cost-effective, given the volume of standardized work they handle and their established networks. They can frequently collaborate with us or your chosen designer to draft an initial plan, rough cost estimates, and a timeline, usually for less than $10,000. Feel free to approach us for guidance on whether this could be a viable option for you.

A WORD OF CAUTION

Be wary of "free" offers, particularly when it comes to plans from dental supply companies. While it may initially seem like they're orchestrating the project on your behalf, there's often a catch: a compulsory purchase of dental equipment, sometimes reaching or exceeding $100,000. Should you opt not to go forward with this mandated equipment purchase, these companies may slap you with a bill for the previously "free" service or, even more frustratingly, withhold the file from your construction team. Such a scenario can lead to significant time and resource wastage. It's also worth noting that the often hefty $100,000 investment might only equip two to three rooms at most. For dentists striving for swift debt clearance, this limited setup may not yield the desired productivity. Moreover, many items included in these premium-priced rooms might not be indispensable for your practice.

PREPARATION IS KEY

Before delving into the realm of permit plans, ensure you've got all your financial ducks in a row:

- Confirm your loan pre-approval

- Lock in lease or purchase terms

- Establish a clear-cut construction budget

- Determine an equipment budget and finalize vendors

By proactively addressing these components, you're laying down a solid foundation to ensure the seamless progression of your dental practice establishment.

VARIABILITY OF CONSTRUCTION COSTS

One of the most unpredictable elements when setting up a dental practice is the construction cost. Several factors contribute to this unpredictability, including regional variations, the contrast between urban and rural areas, prevailing site conditions, the specific scope of work, current demand for contractors and subcontractors, availability of materials, any landlord-provided allowances, and the choice of finishing materials.

A PRACTICAL SCENARIO

To put things in perspective, for a dental practice setup spanning 2,000 sq. ft. with six operational rooms (often referred to as 'ops'), your construction costs will likely fall between $350,000 and $500,000. Remember, this estimate is exclusive of dental equipment costs.

Due to this wide range of factors, providing a standardized or average number is quite challenging. However, for the sake of facilitating a preliminary budget:

GENERAL ESTIMATE

If we consider a typical retail leasehold space, like a unit in a retail plaza or strip mall, construction costs usually hover between $180 and $250 per square foot.

TENANT IMPROVEMENT ALLOWANCES (TIA)

This estimate does not factor in any Tenant Improvement Allowance provided by the landlord. When such allowances are provided, they usually range from $20 to $50 per square foot. More often than not, this allowance manifests as deferred rent. However, it's prudent to be prepared to finance all your expenses independently, without relying heavily on these concessions. For a deeper dive into optimizing your lease, refer to our section titled "Signing the Lease", which provides insights on structuring a mutually beneficial agreement for both the tenant and the landlord.

DENTAL EQUIPMENT

Equipment costs generally range between $15k and $60k per operatory. A budget of $25k-$30k per operatory can lead to a highly efficient workspace, contrary to what you may have been told. Typically, in a startup loan of about $700k, roughly 25% (or $150k-$200k) will be designated for equipment and technology. This budget should adequately outfit 4 to 5 treatment rooms, covering sterilization, the lab, 2D Pan, and mechanicals. For a more in-depth breakdown, refer to our Dental Equipment section.

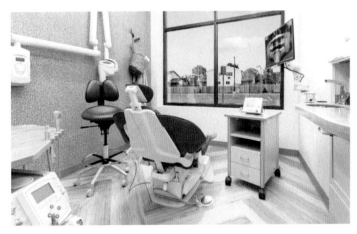

Avoiding bulky side cabinets is a great way to optimize the use of space within your operatories, reduces setup costs, and minimizes the risk of having supplies expire and need to be discarded.

WORKING CAPITAL

Even with top-notch marketing strategies, it might take several months for the cash flow to stabilize. The process of submitting to insurance and then waiting for reimbursement can often span 30 to 60 days. This time frame assumes that the submission was complete, correct, and fully approved...Which you might not do a great job with at first. Moreover, be cautious: some patients might evade payment. These individuals often target new practices.

Until you achieve your initial goals for new patient inflow, production, and collections – whether daily, weekly, or monthly – your practice might operate at a deficit. Although this situation usually lasts no more than three months, we recommend planning for six months. This cautious approach ensures that you don't face cash flow issues early in your startup phase and that the experience for new patients remains uncompromised.

WHEN EQUIPPING YOUR PRACTICE, AVOID THESE PITFALLS:

1. Avoid Bargain Hunting at the Expense of Quality

While everyone loves a deal, remember that "you get what you pay for." Let's consider a scenario where you opt for refurbished patient chairs at $4k each. If one breaks down within three months, you'd face technician fees of around $200/hr plus parts. This first repair could set you back $500-$1,000. On top of that, consider the lost revenue from an unusable chair, potentially amounting to $1,000 or more per day. If such issues persist, a brand-new chair priced at $6,500 with a five-year warranty might soon appear as the wiser investment. (Note: This doesn't imply splurging on a $12k chair right out of the gate. Budgeting is crucial for startups.)

2. Beware of "Free" Deals with Hidden Costs

Some dealers may tempt you with a "free" design model, but there's often a catch. These deals might tie you to room designs costing between $40k-$60k each, limiting you to only 2 or 3 rooms initially. This limited capacity can hinder a new dentist aiming for quick debt clearance. Think of it this way: launching your practice without a hygienist is akin to beginning a race with shoelaces undone. The struggle to maintain patient volume for profitable cash flow would be doubled.

Now, you might wonder what half a year's expenses might amount to. Even though our aim is to keep expenses below average, using the average as a benchmark is prudent. According to the ADA, the average annual expenses for a solo practitioner (excluding the shareholder's salaries) stand at $404k. So, aiming for half of that as a target seems reasonable, with the expectation that the other half will be met through timely payments.

In our experience, having about $200k as working capital is a robust target. However, we understand that not every project or loan package can accommodate this amount. If you can finance this sum yourself, think of it as a valuable insurance policy. To give you a perspective, in our usual $700k startup loan, only about 10% - 15%, which amounts to $70k - $100k, is allocated for working capital. Honestly, that might not give you much peace of mind.

That leads us to a piece of financial advice as you transition into your new practice: consider retaining your associate position for 2-3 days a week. While it might not be what you hoped to hear, it's a prudent financial consideration. Maintaining a stable personal income during this transition period offers an added layer of security, propelling your practice's success. It allows your new venture to evolve naturally, handling challenges without stressing its finances or staff.

Moreover, maintaining a mutually beneficial relationship with another practice has its perks. It can be helpful during times of leave, whether due to vacations or illnesses. Collaborating on complementary clinical skills, referring patients to each other, and sharing training or coaching sessions are just a few benefits. However, if you can't stand your current employer, this might not be a viable solution.

BUSINESS PLAN

A Business Plan isn't just a document lenders ask for—it's a cornerstone of your practice. Every lender will want to review a written Business Plan during the application process. But beyond securing financing, your Business Plan is a reflection of your intentions. It should articulate who you are and your mission.

Your relationship with the business plan shouldn't be passive. Embrace it. Understand its contents, believe in its goals, and be prepared to implement its strategies daily.

While it's essential to cover the basics—like your operating hours, strategies to attract patients, and the type of dentistry you aim to offer—don't overlook the finer points. Incorporate elements such as your Mission Statement, Vision, Impact Diagram, and Core Values. These elements will not only form the backbone of your practice's philosophy but will also guide your marketing initiatives and shape interactions with both patients and staff. Need inspiration? Take a look at our sample Business Plan in the Resources section.

CASH FLOW PROJECTIONS

Cash flow isn't just about numbers—it's the lifeblood of any business. While some lenders might not specifically ask for Cash Flow Projections, preparing one is an invaluable exercise. Remember, businesses thrive or struggle based on cash flow, not just what's reflected on the Profit & Loss statement or the Balance Sheet. With a well-thought-out projection, you can set clear production goals and anticipate how expanding your team, perhaps with hygienists or associate doctors, might boost your revenue.

So, how do you craft a Cash Flow Projection? Start with fundamental metrics like the number of new patients, the number of operational stations (ops), production per op, and the total number of providers. Map these figures onto a 12-month spreadsheet. As you chart each month, estimate how much each provider will contribute to the revenue. As the months progress and you potentially add more providers or utilize more treatment rooms, expect your revenue to rise.

Visualizing this growth and understanding its logic is crucial. After tallying up the total projected revenue, divide this by your monthly rent cost. The resulting percentage should stay below the rent budget you've set for the entire year. While you might find the initial months exceed this limit, increasing production should bring this percentage closer to your target as the year unfolds.

For a practical example, refer to our sample Cash Flow Projection in the Resources section, which illustrates a practice expanding from 4 to 7 chairs.

6 SITE SELECTION & DEMOGRAPHICS

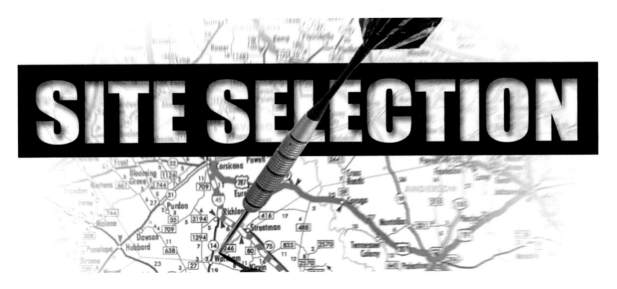

When it comes to startup locations, many practitioners gravitate towards areas popular with young families. Why? Consider this: a single mom, responsible for 85% of household healthcare decisions, could introduce 2-4 potential new patients to your practice. This means one well-executed marketing campaign might connect you with hundreds, even thousands of patients.

However, this is just one approach among many. We've witnessed successful practice launches in diverse locations, from remote oil towns in Canada to bustling downtown Manhattan. Retirement communities, too, can offer promising opportunities. When selecting a site, it's essential to plan for a life where you can cater to your desired clientele, but also to understand and meet the specific needs of the local market.

Navigating site options in booming areas can be daunting. With a range of spaces available, which can differ in price by up to 60%, comparing them is no small feat. Major companies like McDonald's, Kroger, and Walmart have honed their site selection strategies to an art, maximizing their market reach. While they might guard their methodologies closely, it's worth noting that what works for a fast-food giant might not be ideal for a dental practice. Among other distinctions, these large enterprises rely on substantially higher traffic counts to justify their expenditures.

However, there's a silver lining. Recognizing the significance of site selection, we at Design Ergonomics embarked on a mission to develop the industry's most advanced site selector tool. Harnessing the power of contemporary GPS and newly accessible demographic data, we invested over two years in researching and evaluating successful practice locations. The result? A meticulous 100+ point comparative tool that has consistently demonstrated its accuracy.

With this tool, the previously intuitive, (scary), gut-driven decisions that could shape your entire career become data-driven ones. And while countless factors will influence the suitability of each site, we've pinpointed the top six criteria you should prioritize when scouting your first (or next) location.

POPULATION TO DENTIST RATIO

An initial evaluation for any aspiring dental practice involves understanding both the existing dentist count and the local population. You can obtain this information with a straightforward Google search, yielding a general dentist-to-population ratio. Consider the potential challenges of starting your practice within a mile of several other recent and eager dental practices. These newer ventures might share your enthusiasm and readiness to cater to patients' schedules, thereby intensifying competition. Conversely, setting up near a couple of older, more established practices, which might lack aggressive marketing and have limited operating hours, could be advantageous.

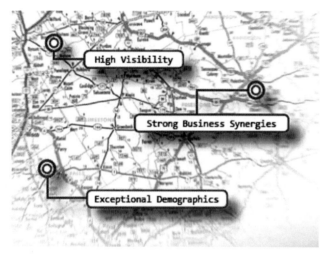

There's a science to finding the right practice location.

A desirable standard ratio is around 2,500:1 for the population to dentist. A lower dentist density can simplify the task of acquiring new patients via marketing. Still, remember that not all dental offices operate on the same level. Your unique marketing strategy, service assortment, operational hours, and office amenities can significantly boost your competitive edge.

AVERAGE HOUSEHOLD – SIZE, INCOME, EDUCATION

Targeting areas with preferable demographics can be particularly beneficial. For instance, if you aim for a family-focused approach, scouting areas with households averaging 4-5 members, boasting above-average incomes (over $75k for dual earners), and higher educational attainment (over 90% high school graduates and 60% with college degrees) might be ideal. Serving such communities often leads to a loyal, multi generational clientele, inclined towards referrals. The influx of referrals can consequently reduce marketing costs and foster higher case acceptance.

To assess potential locales, utilize resources like city-data.com, census.gov, and incomedatabyzipcode.com. These platforms offer insights into regions that match your desired patient profile.

TRAFFIC COUNT & VISIBILITY

A general guideline in this domain is a 1000:1 car-to-new patient ratio per day. For a goal of 100 new patients monthly, with a 20-day operational month (implying 5 new patients daily), the target would be a minimum of 5,000 car passersby daily. However, higher traffic is always preferable.

Many states offer transportation department websites that furnish data on major roadway traffic counts, and more tailored information might be available upon request. But exercise caution; elevated traffic doesn't guarantee a rise in new patients. While generally, more traffic is favorable, several other nuanced factors play a role in the site-selection procedure.

For practices in densely populated urban areas like New York, Boston, L.A., or San Francisco, other factors take precedence. Proximity to public transit systems becomes critical. Modern urban planning now emphasizes "walkability"—the ease of navigating areas on foot, focusing on proper sidewalks, crosswalks, pedestrian bridges, and roads. If most of your patients are pedestrians or users of public transport, it's advisable to select locations within close reach of major residential zones.

ACCESSIBILITY

Accessibility reflects the ease with which patients can travel from their homes or workplaces to your dental practice. Consider the major routes and roads leading to your establishment.

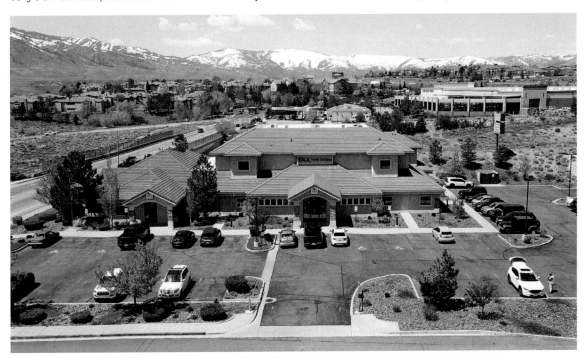

Sala Family Dentistry understands the importance of convenient parking and a clearly identifiable patient entrance.

What kind of traffic patterns do they encounter? Is your parking area or plaza entrance easily accessible? Are there recognizable signs or landmarks guiding them? Once they arrive, is it straightforward to find a parking spot and make their way into your facility?

This isn't just a concern from a marketing perspective; while you certainly don't want to squander advertising efforts on attracting new patients who find it challenging to reach you, it's also essential for operational efficiency. Imagine targeting an audience that's separated from your location by a river or train tracks. Traffic congestion near your establishment due to inadequate road designs, traffic lights, or entry and exit points can frequently cause patients to be late. This can significantly disrupt your daily schedule, compromising patient experience, affecting staff morale, and potentially impacting your daily productivity. It might mean the difference between completing a crown procedure in one appointment or having to reschedule, or missing out on an additional procedure discovered during a routine checkup.

PARKING

Parking is an often underestimated aspect when choosing a site for a new dental practice. As a benchmark, aim for 1 to 1.5 parking spots for every treatment room designated for patients, and an additional parking space for each full-time employee. To illustrate, if an average dental office has 5 treatment rooms – comprising 2 operative rooms, 2 hygiene rooms, and one overflow room – the staffing might include 2 assistants, 2 hygienists, and 2 administrative personnel for each dentist. This configuration alone necessitates 7 parking spots solely for staff in a single-doctor practice. Adding the patient parking requirement only amplifies the need.

For a larger setup, such as a 10-chair facility with two dentists, approximately 15 parking spots would be required for patients and an additional 10-15 for employees. That totals to a substantial 30 parking spaces for a two-dentist establishment. Overlooking this critical aspect could jeopardize the appeal and functionality of your location.

7 OFFICE DESIGN

Discussing all the various types of practices one can design would be exhaustive. Each type has its unique criteria, opportunities, and challenges. However, it's worth noting that over 70% of startups involve general dentists setting up their first practice in burgeoning urban or suburban areas. Hence, for the sake of this guide, we'll view the topic from this angle.

When diving into the design process, it's crucial to consider the future. Ask yourself: where do you envision your practice in the next 3-5 years? This foresight is essential since, on average, it takes that long for a practice to reach full capacity (2-3 restorative and 2-3 hygiene columns being 80%+ booked two weeks in advance). Once you hit that capacity (and chances are, you'll do so quicker than anticipated with proper management planning), what's your next step?

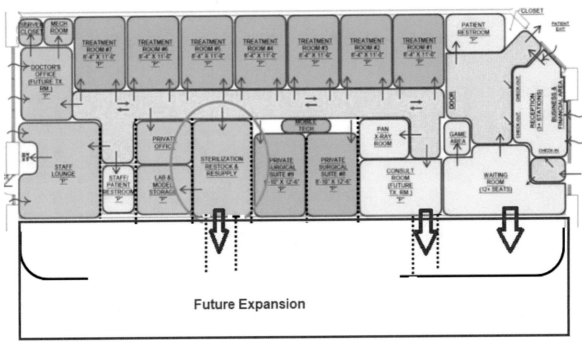

An example plan that would permit easy expansion to the adjacent space.

Expanding an office can be an excellent investment. Such an expansion can benefit from the infrastructure and systems set up during the initial setup. Naturally, with increased demand, there's a need for more providers. Its important to secure "first right of refusal" to adjacent spaces in your lease when possible. See chapter 7 for more information.

Every doctor requires treatment rooms, and these rooms necessitate space. But how much space is adequate?

In the U.S., the typical general dentist operates from 5 treatment rooms: 2 for hygiene, 2 for the doctor, and 1 overflow room for immediate needs or emergencies. This model has proven effective and provides ample opportunity to generate over $1M annually from dentistry alone.

More ambitious doctors, or those in states with accommodating laws for dental assistants, may even operate from up to 7 rooms: 3 for hygiene, 3 for restorative treatments, and 1 overflow. Such a setup not only ups the ante but also simplifies the process of introducing an associate doctor later on. For the context of this guide, let's use the 5-room model as our baseline. However, remember, it's flexible and can be increased if needed should your vision be more ambitious.

Finally, to determine the ideal building size, multiply the total number of treatment rooms by a specific ratio. This ratio is influenced by how you plan to outfit your treatment rooms and the efficiency of your operational process. While you might not be mulling over this now, it's a detail that deserves your attention before moving forward. Both room layout and process flow are equally important.

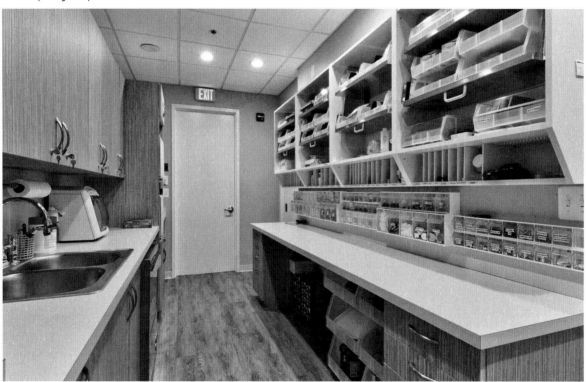

The resupply area creates a centralized hub for dental office clinical support. A great example of visual restocking and use of vertical space with hydraulic PullDown™ cabinetry.

OFFICE CENTRIC VS. ROOM CENTRIC DESIGNS

In modern office layouts, two types of treatment room designs stand out: one that integrates substantial storage within each room, typically as side cabinetry, and another that does not. The former is termed "Room Centric" design, while the latter is known as "Office Centric" design.

As detailed in the chapter dedicated to this topic in our Blueprint to Maximizing Productivity, any dental office anticipating expansion beyond 3 or 4 treatment rooms should primarily consider the Office Centric design. This recommendation stems from two key reasons: Cost and Production Efficiency.

The Room Centric design tends to incorporate larger spaces, sometimes measuring up to 10' x 12'. These extensive dimensions can consume a significant portion of the office's total area. Moreover, such a design doesn't necessarily align with the evolving requirements of contemporary dentistry, which demand versatile procedural setups and adaptable scheduling. When viewed from both a doctor's and an assistant's standpoint, these large rooms actually necessitate more time and effort to complete similar tasks, invariably leading to reduced productivity.

On the other hand, the Office Centric design champions more streamlined rooms, typically in the 9'x11' range. Here, only the supplies required for 1-2 weeks of procedures are stored in-room. The remaining inventory is centralized in a primary sterilization area, which functions as the office's core, with the treatment rooms branching out like spokes. This approach, reminiscent of a manufacturing model aptly dubbed "One Piece Flow" in Toyota terminology, offers a slew of advantages:

1. Significant reduction in supply costs.

2. Considerably faster room setup and turnaround time.

3. Enhanced ergonomic movements and accessibility for both the doctor and assistant.

4. A more spacious and welcoming ambiance for patients, contrasting the sometimes congested appearance created by side cabinetry. (For a deeper dive into the impact of space on psychology, visit https://desergo.com/blog/the-psychology-of-space-when-designing-a-dental-office)

ROOM YIELD

In terms of size ratios, Office Centric office designs require about 330 sq. ft. per treatment room, while Room Centric ones need roughly 450 sq. ft. Therefore, envisioning a 10-treatment room practice serving two doctors, you'd need a space close to 3,300 sq. ft. with an Office Centric approach, as opposed to 4,500 sq. ft. for a Room Centric configuration. Planning for potential expansion is wise. This foresight can be achieved by requesting "First Right of Refusal" clauses be added to the lease for any adjoining spaces or by obtaining the required square footage and leaving it undeveloped until patient demand justifies its use, more on this is covered in the next chapter. (If you're lucky enough to have a freestanding building, ensure there's ample space on the property for future growth.)

Before delving into the design process, it's crucial to understand the concept of Room Yield. This term, which is originates in the way retailers view the value of a property, serves as a swift metric to determine the efficiency of potential and existing practices. To compute it, take the total square footage of a building and divide it by the number of Treatment Rooms.

For instance, take three different practices, each with 10 treatment rooms (ops). If one is 3,000 sq. ft., the second is 4,250 sq. ft., and the third is 5,000 sq. ft., their room yields would be 300 sq. ft./op, 425 sq. ft./op, and 500 sq. ft./op, respectively. This provides a rough indication of the productive capacity per square foot achieved by the initial design. Decreasing OR increasing this too much will reduce performance! Both initial construction cost and ongoing maintenance expenses are largely determined by the total square footage of a building. Hence, achieving a favorable yield during the initial design phase is critical.

We've found that a yield of approximately 330 sq. ft./op is an ideal benchmark in most design scenarios for startup practices. Yields lower than this might indicate a shortage of amenities for patients or staff, such as break rooms, administrative workstations, restrooms, and waiting areas. This is not to suggest that lower figures are unattainable, but achieving them may necessitate specialized design expertise, specific practice management approaches, and certain geometric considerations. On the other hand, a yield exceeding this benchmark might indicate inefficiencies in the design, such as oversized treatment rooms, excessive or expansive hallways, or unproductive administrative and office spaces. It's noteworthy that the industry average, as indicated by the many dental supply company plans that come across our desk, hovers around 450 sq. ft./op. For a 10-op office, this translates to an extra 800 sq. ft. for the same productive capacity. At a construction cost of $200 per sq. ft., this could mean an added $160,000 in expenses! As highlighted in the Finance section, construction is the most significant and challenging cost to mitigate in the entire project.

To put this into perspective, that extra cost could equip 4-5 additional treatment rooms!

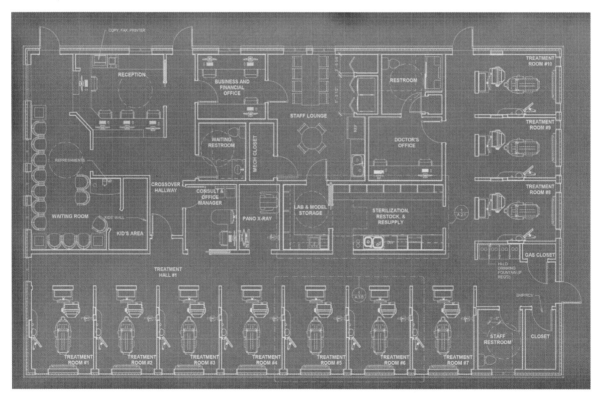

An example dental office floor plan.

18 ELEMENTS OF AN IDEAL OFFICE DESIGN

With over three decades exclusively designing dental offices. Design Ergonomics has identified a set of vital features that distinguish a mediocre office design from a good one, and a good design from an exceptional one. For a comprehensive list with detailed explanations and examples, visit the "18 Elements Codified" in our Resources section.

By referencing this list and evaluating your design against it, you'll ensure your space is not only functional but also comfortable, efficient, and productive. Adhering to these guidelines heightens the likelihood that patients will have an outstanding experience that you will become highly productive, and that the staff will benefit from an environment tailored specifically to facilitate their work. Deviating from these principles will be to your detriment!

Please Note: The features mentioned pertain to architectural elements. In addition to these, interior design elements play a pivotal role. If you need guidance on crafting an emotionally resonant interior, refer to our article titled "18 Elements of an Ideal Interior Design" available on our website.

ATTRACT & IMPRESS PATIENTS	1. Clearly identifiable patient entrance 2. Staff entrance screened from view 3. Immediate visual and physical access to the front desk upon entering the reception area
KEEP PATIENTS RELAXED	4. Reception area seating ("patient lounge") removed from primary circulation or traffic flow 5. Patient bathroom visible to, but removed from, the patient lounge 6. The major proportion of the open front desk does not face the patient lounge 7. Treatment rooms isolated from the front desk 8. Consultation room location minimally exposes patients to treatment room activities 9. Consultation room accessible by the doctor without passing into the patient lounge or front desk space 10. Treatment room alignment does not channel noises from room to room
CREATE A NATURAL FLOW FOR PROCESSES	11. Sterilization, lab, and resupply areas in close physical proximity to treatment rooms 12. Treatment rooms should be spacious, but space-efficient, maximizing both productivity and patient comfort 13. Compact treatment area minimizing segregation of doctor and hygiene staff 14. Doctor's office within proximity of treatment rooms, permitting doctor to keep a pulse on clinical activities 15. Space for mobilization of technology 16. Imaging areas do not block traffic flow when in use 17. Staff lounge isolated from clinical and business zones 18. Office expansion easily accommodated with minimal practice disruption

CONCERNS & LIMITATIONS IN THE DESIGN PROCESS

Every ideal office design comes with its own set of challenges. Often, these stem from architectural or structural features that either can't be moved or would be too expensive to alter. These might include structural columns and support beams, CMU/Brick walls or partitions, variations in interior floor height, electrical and gas meter panels, utility chases that sometimes serve other floors or units, ground-mounted HVAC units, bank vaults, and more.

Although these factors shouldn't deter you from considering a potential location, it's crucial to obtain an accurate "As Built" plan early in any due diligence phase. This ensures that every element is recognized, allowing your designer to strategize on addressing any uncovered constraints.

Unexpected discoveries, like a structural column or utility chase during demolition, can stall a project. Such unforeseen obstacles can necessitate a complete floor plan redesign, especially if they emerge in a problematic spot.

Paying for an builder for the "As Built" service is a wise investment. This foresight not only prevents potential roadblocks but also ensures that the individuals identifying the issues are the ones responsible for resolving them. This dynamic leads to swift evaluations of cost versus benefit scenarios and available options. It's also why we highly advocate for the design-build construction approach whenever possible—it streamlines the development process, addressing potential problems early on.

OWN VS. LEASE

While the choice to own or lease may not significantly influence the design, it's worth noting that leasing can come with certain constraints. These might relate to construction specifications, aesthetic guidelines, permitted construction hours, and building access. Such potential limitations should be clarified before finalizing a lease agreement.

Other factors to consider include the landlord's openness to modifying windows and doors, creating new exterior openings, addressing property deficiencies (like wheelchair accessibility), and sorting out any service or utility issues.

Engage in candid discussions with the property owner or their representatives well in advance of your intended changes. Seek their input and approval. It's vital to get these agreements documented and incorporated into the lease agreement, as appropriate.

If the landlord or their representatives seem reluctant or unresponsive to such collaboration, treat it as a cautionary sign and explore other leasing opportunities.

ARCHITECTS, MEPS & PERMITS

After finalizing the initial design, developing the floor plan, agreeing on the lease terms, and securing financial pre-approvals, it's time to proceed with the necessary plans for obtaining construction permits.

Each state licenses architects and professional engineers who are mandated to draft these plans and offer their formal approval. Once these plans receive a stamp of approval, they can be presented to the Building Department for permits. Once granted, the General Contractor retrieves the plans and permits, paving the way for construction to begin.

"MEPs" refer to Mechanical, Electrical, and Plumbing plans, which typically encompass:

- HVAC System Size and Configuration

- Electrical load assessments, panel dimensions, and circuit diagrams.

- Layouts for domestic water supply and drainage.

- Life safety provisions and fire escape strategies.

- Reviews of ADA accessibility and code compliance.

- Necessary structural engineering.

Should you choose a Design-Build firm, this aspect will be integrated into the comprehensive package provided by the builder, eliminating the need to address it as a separate project component.

INTERIOR DESIGN

A common oversight we notice in startup planning is a disconnect between the floor plan design and the actual aesthetic of the office — the Interior Design.

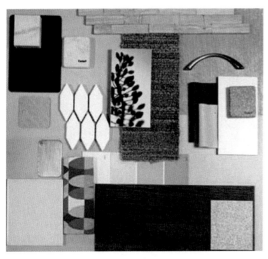

Creating a "Design Board" is a fun and effective way to think through detailed design choices for your practice.

This discrepancy often arises because many doctors, aiming to ensure that their selected space meets functional needs, opt for a free office plan from whoever will provide it. However, a dealer's primary objective is to sell equipment, not to craft an integral component of your long-term success plan. Moreover, these dealers cater to numerous offices in your area. Are they truly best suited to help you uniquely express yourself through your office's design and guarantee that your practice stands out as the best in town? Think of it this way, they are helping build a new office that competes with their golfing buddy! Your commitment is to yourself, aiming to build the finest office within your budget. It's crucial to cultivate a design that genuinely resonates with your target clientele, even if it diverges from your personal preferences! Here's the crux: achieving this vision necessitates an interior designer's expertise to ensure that:

1. Your clients are enamored with the design. (You want them to rave to all their friends!)

2. The aesthetic complements the planned architectural layout.

3. The design employs durable yet cost-effective materials, balancing appearance and longevity.

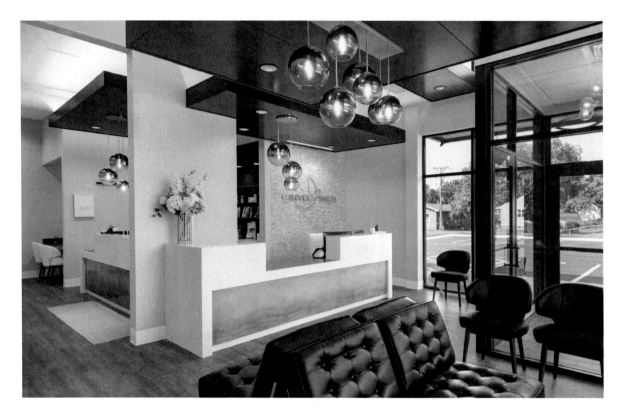

Contractors often lack this aesthetic finesse. Surprisingly, architects might not be specifically trained in this either. And as an individual, despite binge-watching HGTV, your knowledge in this domain is probably more limited than you think. Save that budding design passion for your future dream home, funded by your flourishing practice, and let professionals excel in their specialty. We've witnessed enough DIY mishaps to advise otherwise.

Embark on your Interior Design journey soon after locking in a space, and definitely before finalizing the Floor Plan and MEPs. For instance, determining the contour of your reception desk should be influenced by your broader style vision. Are you leaning towards crisp modern lines or gentler curves? Wood and stone, or steel and glass? Neo-Colonial or Modern Chic? Each choice can impact the layout itself. It's crucial to ensure your meticulously crafted plan aligns with the aesthetic preferences of both you and your clients. You can't just put lipstick on it when it's done.

Upon finalizing a style and ensuring the floor plan embodies it, the comprehensive Interior Design Plan will emerge. This plan details finish and material choices, lighting, bathroom fixtures, furniture, ceiling plans, interior elevations, and more. These details are paramount for accurate construction estimates, providing contractors with a clear blueprint of required materials and construction techniques. The clearer the plan, the more accurate the cost estimates!

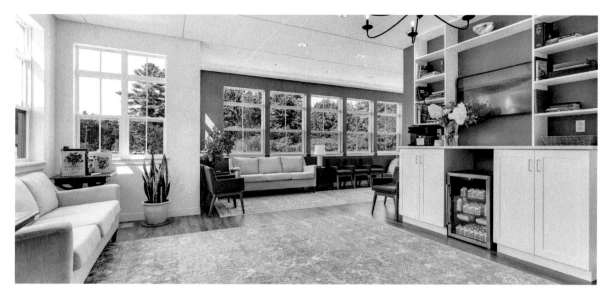

Here's a concise checklist of materials and specifications you'll need to decide upon:

- General and accent paint colors.

- Materials for counter tops and work surfaces.

- Specifications for cabinet construction, including type, material, and colors.

- Door and window details.

- Selections for hardware such as hinges, doorknobs, drawer handles, etc.

- Types, materials, and transitions of flooring.

- Specifications for bathroom and kitchen fixtures and appliances.

- Details for general, task, and decorative lighting fixtures, as well as their placements.

- Choices for artwork and furniture.

An adept interior designer considers both aesthetics and functionality, ensuring the space caters to all five senses from the perspectives of patients and staff. This encompasses visual appeal, optimal sightlines, ensuring pleasant (or neutral) scents, curating ambient background music, minimizing clinical noises, and even tactile experiences like furniture and amenities. Taste may also be considered, particularly when offering refreshments or facilities like brushing/rinsing stations. Simply put, interior design isn't just about appearance; it's a pivotal component of your brand's identity.

Clearly, decisions in this domain profoundly influence both the budget and project timeline. It's crucial for your designer and builder to maintain open lines of communication throughout the process. This ensures that any design decisions or modifications are swiftly integrated into the overarching cost and schedule.

IT AND TECHNOLOGY

During the MEP phase, it's essential to finalize the technology infrastructure for your new practice. Here's a list of key decisions you'll need to make:

- **Cloud vs. Server-Based**
  Will your data be stored on the cloud or on an on-premises server?

- **Connectivity**
  Do you prefer hardwired connections or Wi-Fi?

- **Computing Devices**
  Are you leaning towards desktops or laptops for your workspace?

- **Security**
  Are you considering installing a sound and security system? (Hint: You probably should!)

- **Software**
  Which practice management and imaging software will best serve your needs?

- **Payment Processing**
  Have you decided on a credit card processing company?

- **Printing**
  What will you need to print, and where will the printers be located?

- **Communication**
  What phone system do you plan to adopt? Are you considering tracking or recording calls? Additionally, will you need an after-hours phone or answering service?

Each of these considerations may involve specialized expertise. It's crucial to engage with professionals who have experience in setting up dental offices, especially for startups. They can guide you in distinguishing the "Must-Haves" from the "Nice-to-Haves." While some elements might be postponed for future incorporation, it's vital to ensure that the initial setup can accommodate any foundational infrastructure they might require.

Remember, it's the little detailing like data jacks and power outlets that can make a difference. Installing these while the framing is still exposed is both easy and cost-effective. However, once the walls are up and painted, making these additions becomes both costly and disruptive.

8 SIGNING THE LEASE

Before we proceed with signing a lease, it's crucial to draft one. The contents of this lease will predominantly stem from your initial Letter of Intent and the subsequent responses from the landlord. For your reference, we've incorporated a Sample Letter of Intent in the Resources section. You may wish to engage a professional lease negotiator to help you with this, more on that later in this chapter.

Interestingly, dentists are regarded as one of the most reliable commercial tenants. They boast among the lowest default rates among all small businesses. Moreover, they often commit to longer-than-average leases, spanning 10 years or more. Such tenures can uplift both the value and the image of the building and its neighboring area. Given these advantages, it's imperative to remember that accepting the landlord's initial offer without any negotiation is not advisable. Always strive to negotiate terms that are in your favor.

Consider this: over a term of 10 or more years for a 3,000 sq. ft. space, a dentist might end up paying an amount ranging from $500k to $1M in rent. From this perspective, it seems entirely reasonable to request considerations like six months of deferred rent for construction or an allowance of $50 per sq. ft. for tenant build-outs. Even if this means paying a slightly higher rent per square foot, the upfront capital savings makes it a sound decision in the long run.

The sample lease provided sheds light on several components, including:

- A description of the property.

- The type of lease (single, double, or triple NET).

- Lease duration and extension possibilities.

- Rent amount and potential increases.

- Numerous legal provisions detailing responsibilities for repairs, maintenance, snow removal, and so forth.

However, there are four particular aspects of the lease that merit focused negotiation:

SIGNAGE

Your signage's location and size can be powerful tools for marketing, as outlined in our subsequent Marketing section. It's crucial to push for the most sizable, prominent, and easily visible sign permissible. Many landlords might restrict you to the standard monument sign shared with other tenants in the parking lot. However, certain locations, especially corner suites or standalone units, might offer the option to affix your sign directly to the building. Such positioning can amplify your sign's visibility tenfold. Remember, a strategically placed sign often provides one of the best returns on investment in marketing.

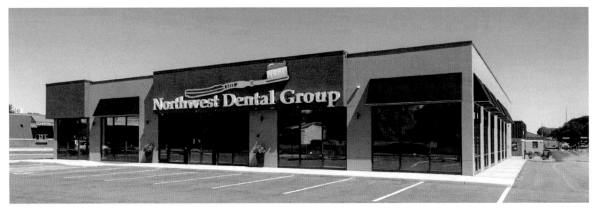

The toothbrush sign at Northwest Dental Group is fun and eye-catching.

ASSIGNMENT

One essential clause is the "Assignment of Lease." This provision allows you to transfer all the rights held by the lessee (tenant) concerning the property to another party. While this is a standard clause and shouldn't be an issue for landlords, it can sometimes be overlooked. With this provision in your lease, selling your business becomes seamless as you can include the assets and the lease in the sale. In its absence, you'd need to negotiate with the landlord to confirm they're willing to draft a new lease for the prospective buyer. You'd also find yourself potentially mediating between the buyer and the landlord to settle on favorable rates. This could be a complicated situation, which the Assignment clause conveniently sidesteps.

FIRST RIGHT OF REFUSAL

Another significant clause is the "First Right of Refusal." This provision ensures that the tenant gets priority to lease any available spaces adjacent to theirs. Most startup dental practices in North America typically find the need to expand within their initial five years of operation. Refer to our "Math of Growth" article for a detailed explanation on the pace and scale of this growth. However, in our experience, over 75% of the startups we've engaged with have required this expansion, including those on their second or third ventures with 10 to 15 operations. With this clause, you're essentially reserving potential expansion space that would be otherwise unattainable without moving to a new location. If you're considering a retail location with several available spaces, it might be strategic to choose spaces adjacent to businesses that have higher turnover rates. Examples of such businesses include barber shops, nail salons, pet groomers, martial arts studios, and smaller restaurants. This contrasts with low turnover establishments like big box stores, chain restaurants, supermarkets, liquor stores, and convenience stores.

ALLOWANCES AND DEFERRALS

The third crucial area pertains to the Tenant Improvement Allowance (often referred to as "TI money") and the terms of rent deferral. As previously discussed, a lease spanning 10 years with options for multiple 5-year extensions can equate to almost $1M in rental income for the landlord. Hence, requesting allowances like $50 per sq. ft. in TI money or a rent deferment until your business opens isn't an unreasonable demand. Given the minimal impact on the landlord's overall earnings from the lease, it's vital to negotiate this section diligently. If necessary, consider seeking expert assistance to ensure you're positioned favorably.

There are several commercial realtors and lease negotiators who specialize in the dental industry. Carr Realty and George Vail are two who have proven valuable to our clients. However, it's essential to note that they often charge based on a percentage of the rent saved or a pre-agreed amount. This can be somewhat costly upfront because you're essentially covering a percentage of the savings for the entire lease duration at the outset. For instance, if they charge 10% of the saved amount and manage to negotiate your rent down by $4 per sq. ft. from an initial $25/ft rate, that's a saving of $10,000 for a 2,500 sq. ft. space annually. Over a decade, this amounts to $100,000. Thus, their fee could be $10,000 payable upon signing. It's not to suggest that such a fee is unreasonable, but it's vital to be aware of and prepared for this expense if you choose to engage professional services.

Our final piece of advice concerning the lease is straightforward: Don't hesitate to WALK AWAY. Numerous potential locations could suit your next practice, and the available options might differ six months down the line. Rushing into a decade-long agreement is unwise, especially since signing a lease is one of the earliest and most impactful irreversible decisions in this venture. If any aspect feels off—the numbers, lease terms, design, or any other factor—WALK AWAY. You can always explore other spaces, continue saving, reduce your debts, or consider reapplying for a loan later on. Opportunities will keep arising. We recognize the eagerness to start immediately, but we've seen the repercussions of haste. We strongly urge patience and due diligence.

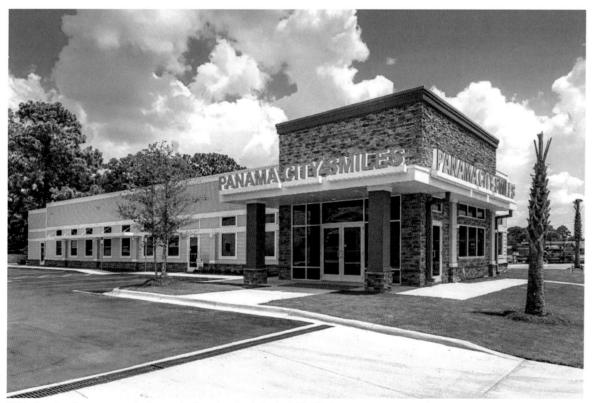

Within the rules of your area, create signage that is on-brand and clearly visible. This is an opportunity to stand out.

9 HIGH PERFORMANCE DENTISTRY

Somewhere within your desire to have your very own dental practice lies the wish to have greater economic success, more free time and less stress. There may be other laudable goals as part of your vision. To be the best implant or Invisalign or preventative doctor for example. All great primary reasons for becoming a dentist in the first place! But nobody makes this effort without the goal of a better quality of life. Here is the crazy part however!

Virtually no dentists know how to do this well! In 2024 the average dentist produces a little over $400.00 per hour. That is horrible! And it also means that half of the dentists produce less than this. This is totally unacceptable, unnecessary and will never provide prosperity!

So before we discuss equipment we must talk about what principles need to be met in order to be highly productive. This will only be a brief overview. Read "Your blueprint for maximizing productivity"Here goes!

1. You can't use what you can't reach.

Humans do dentistry and humans have a circumscribed range of motion. Only seven to 10% of a typical dental appointment is handpiece on tooth time. That is because far too much of the time is actually...not doing dentistry. The time is spent going and getting and setting up and breaking down and deciding what instrument to use and hopefully having it... And all of the reaching and turning and positioning to make that happen! You need a system of production that permits seamless productivity for all of your procedures without twisting, turning or "go and it gets". In order to do that you need five to seven square feet of workspace that is accessible to both doctor and dental assistant. This is impossible to do with side or rear delivery and only possible with an over the patient arrangement if, in addition, you add at least five square feet of support in the assistant over the head position. Remember, in dental school, you really only learn to do one procedure at a time! In practice your patients are begging you to get their work done quickly and comfortably. They don't actually want you to produce not much and do it slowly!

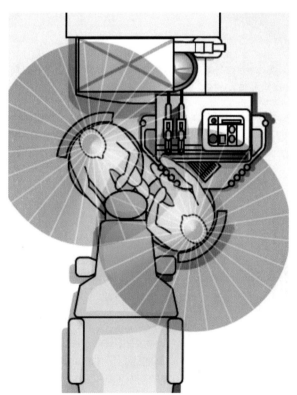

You can't use what you can't reach!

2. You need a plan to centralize all of your supplies and not hide them in a storage closet but also not have them out where they look ugly to the patient. Toyota calls this "visual restocking".

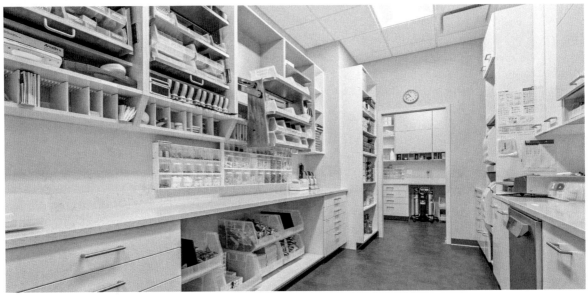

Visual restocking in a centralized resupply area.

3. Sterilization should be located where restocking is done. Toyota has a name for this as well. It's called "one piece flow".

4. You will have some technology that you will only own one of. You need a plan for where to mobilize these. As a practices range of technology increases so does the need for mobility planning.

These are the principles that the most productive manufacturers on earth have built in their companies upon. Build your foundation on these as well.

● THREE DECADES OF RESEARCH

In the pursuit of optimal productivity and patient well-being doctor Ahearn and his researchers have spent over three decades evaluating systems for surgical and manufacturing success. This included some rather interesting outliers in the world of surgery including Dr. Svyatoslav Fyodorov who in 1985 with a team of four other surgeons in Russia invented a system to perform over 1000 glaucoma and cataract surgeries a day. At a cost that was at that time less than that of eyeglasses.

Hey, it was Russia in the 1980's. It was that or blindness for many of these patients! But the principles of productivity are immutable. Become a student of them!

10 SELECTING EQUIPMENT FOR A START-UP PRACTICE

Planning your first practice can feel like being a kid in a toy store. The vast array of emerging technologies is both exciting and distracting. New doctors often fall for the sales pitch that claims, "Just a few procedures each month will cover the cost of this product!"

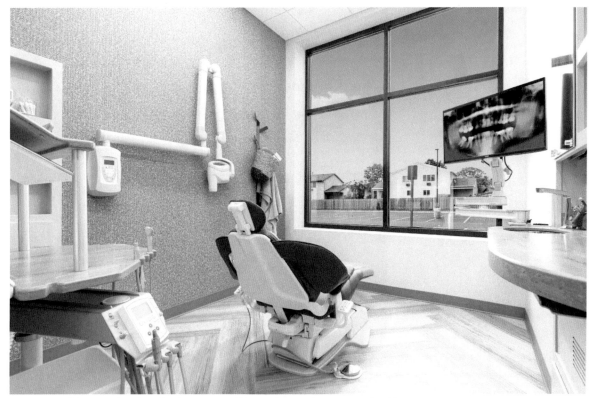

Consider dental delivery options that will make you more efficient and your patients more comfortable.

While we're enthusiastic supporters of advancing technology, succumbing to this allure too early in your practice can strain your budget. Don't fret – there'll be an opportunity for that cutting-edge (CBCT unit) in the future! For now, prioritize products and systems that let you conduct basic dentistry as efficiently and productively as possible. This approach paves the way for growth – leading you to all the high-tech equipment you covet.

When deciding on equipment for a startup, center your attention on three main aspects: bolstering essential performance, trimming labor needs, and increasing the success of case acceptance. The term "essential" is pivotal here. The bulk of your earnings will derive from a standard set of treatments you perform daily. HINT: They are the ones that your new patients actually want! In our Productivity Guide, we term this your "90% Procedure Profile." Choose equipment that enhances efficiency, speed, and comfort for these procedures. Although high-end technologies offer fresh avenues, such treatments will remain outliers at first.

Trimming labor inherently bolsters productivity in treatment. Here, we're referencing labor in a broader sense: not merely the time spent on a specific procedure, but all the auxiliary tasks your team undertakes. Curbing labor expenses is vital during the nascent phases of your practice. Sure, you'll have a loan to offset fixed expenses, but once construction ends, there's a 4-6 month window to rev up cash flow! Given that payroll will be your largest expense during this phase, it's crucial to limit its impact. Clawing your way out from under a hefty, unyielding payroll can be a years-long endeavor. You'll manage, but thriving becomes an uphill battle if you aren't disciplined! If you design your foundational systems to maximize efficiency from day one, you'll liberate resources, positioning your practice for rapid and profitable growth.

OPERATORY EQUIPMENT

Typical treatment rooms are furnished with eight pivotal pieces of equipment:

1. Delivery Unit

2. Headwall Setup

3. Doctor Sidewall

4. Patient + Team Seating

5. Assistant Sidewall

6. Intraoral Dental Light

7. Nitrous Oxide Delivery

8. Imaging Solutions

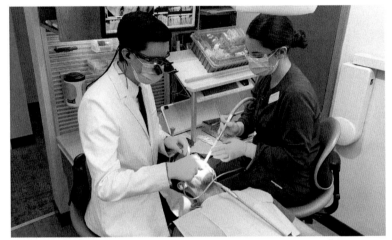

Efficient 4-handed dentistry will make dentistry easier and more efficient. It also elevates the skills of dental assistants leading to greater performance and staff retention.

Each of these tools plays a significant role in patient care. However, some of them, either through labor efficiency or improved performance, substantially enhance productivity from the outset. Recognize and assess this impact while setting your budget, and prioritize equipment that offers immediate top-tier performance. For clarity, we'll categorize these items based on their immediate productivity influence: High and Low.

Delivery Unit
HIGH IMPACT

This stands out as the quintessential equipment in any treatment room. A stellar delivery unit does more than merely house your handpieces. It meticulously organizes every fundamental component required for effective dentistry in a 3D platform, ensuring everything is within arm's reach for both you and your assistant. For optimized efficiency, its proximity to the patient's mouth should be as close as feasible. To conceive a dental treatment room in its essence. The core is the delivery system and a chair!

When we speak of "essential components for dentistry," we're referring to:

- Consumable and operative supplies
- Keyboard and data access
- Medical waste and sharps disposal containers
- Trash bins
- Instrument trays & bur block holders
- Handpieces
- Assistant utilities
- Auxiliary tools like curing lights, scalers, intraoral cameras, and more

Ensuring immediate accessibility to all of these items for both doctors and assistants significantly accelerates procedures. As alluded to previously, the actual procedure duration, or 'time-on-tooth', constitutes a minor amount of the treatment time. Therefore, an exceptional delivery system must cater to every other aspect of the treatment process.

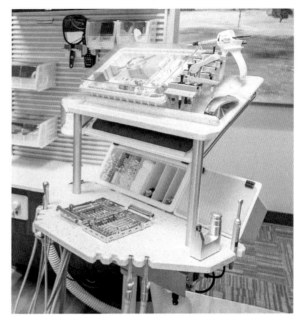

Your delivery unit should function seamlessly during both 2-handed and 4-handed operations. This efficiency cuts down procedure durations and effectively boosts productivity by freeing up appointment slots. Such versatility also facilitates prompt handling of emergency cases and provides adaptability for left-handed/right-handed operators.

Think of this as the linchpin of your productivity. Being the revenue engine of your practice, compromising on the delivery system is inadvisable. Never sacrifice perpetual efficiency, potentially worth $200, $400, or even $800 per hour, to merely save $5,000 upfront. Such savings may appear beneficial in the short run but carry a steep long-term price tag.

TARGET COST
$8,000 - $12,000

Headwall Setup
HIGH IMPACT

Acting as a backbone to your delivery unit, the headwall establishes the primary connection point for all your dental utilities, coupled with providing extra storage and a functional staging area. Often, there's a need for an accessible spot to keep additional procedure kits during treatment such as whitening or implant tubs. The headwall generally hosts the primary computer and monitor for tasks like charting, note-taking, and scheduling all discreetly placed away from the patient's sight in compliance with HIPAA regulations.

Additionally, the headwall becomes a repository for items unnecessary in a 4-handed setup but indispensable when assistants or hygienists are operating solo. This includes items like x-ray sensors, USB ports, polishing tips, prophy pastes, appointment reminder cards, and more. Remember: Hygienists utilizes rooms differently. The room often functions as an office within an office.

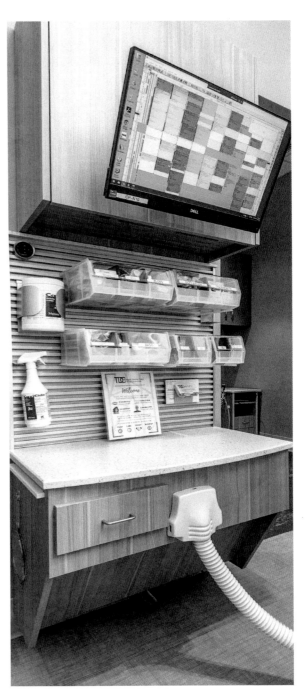

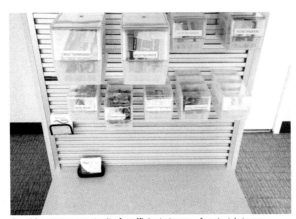

Consider every opportunity for efficient storage of materials in your operatories. Slatwalls with clear storage bins provide vertical storage options and free up space on counters.

TARGET COST

$2,000 - $3,000

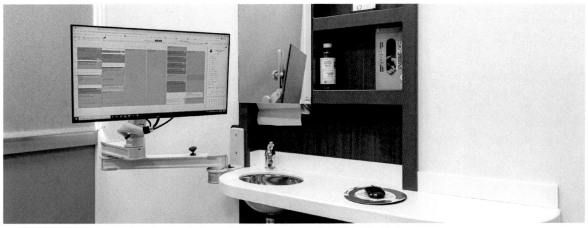

Get rid of bulky side cabinets and use the space between studs for elegant and efficient in-wall cabinetry.

Doctor Sidewall
HIGH IMPACT

The doctor sidewall, when tailored with an extendable monitor, becomes the perfect setting for in-operatory case presentations. Imagine sitting shoulder-to-shoulder with a patient, collaboratively reviewing x-rays and intraoral images for a clearer, holistic, and effective presentation. Equipping it with a payment mechanism (like a credit card reader) amplifies its utility. The entire process—from presenting treatments to scheduling appointments—can be done seamlessly without needing to relocate the patient. This fosters efficient office flow, minimizes handoffs, and curtails employee labor. (For an illustrative guide, view our Case Presentation video.)

Considering adding sinks to your operatories? The doctor sidewall is the optimal place. However, while they're handy, they fall under "nice" rather than "essential". With the delivery unit providing water for alginates, the convenience of hand sanitizers, and patients being able to rinse using a saliva ejector, the pressing need for sinks diminishes in the mind of some. Yet, sinks in rooms offer a touch of care, allowing patients to freshen up post-procedure, enhancing their overall experience. As a tip: a patient's likelihood of accepting a major treatment plan may be directly proportional to their comfort level. If budget permits, it's worth including sinks.

TARGET COST

$2,000 - $4,000

(The higher end of the spectrum incorporating media & sink.)

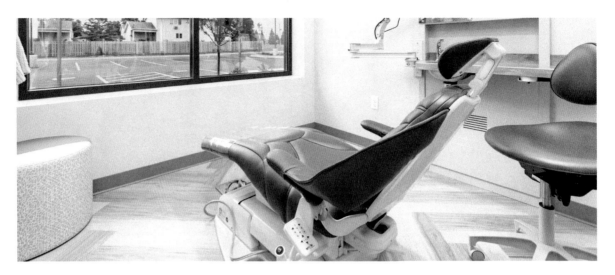

Patient Chair
LOW IMPACT

Your patient is likely to spend the majority of their time in your practice in this chair. Thus, the importance of a chair in enhancing the patient's overall experience cannot be understated. However, it has been categorized as low impact due to:

Non-Immediate Production Impact
While a premium chair can undoubtedly elevate the patient's comfort level, its direct influence on production is subtle. A more comfortable patient might be more inclined towards accepting treatments, but such a chair upgrade can be deferred to a later phase.

Replace-ability Factor
Patient chairs, especially those that aren't tethered with chair-mounted delivery systems, are relatively easy to replace. They can be transitioned in and out of rooms with minimal fuss. Moreover, the availability of refurbished chairs at nearly half the price offers an economical yet functional alternative for the startup practice.

In the vast market of patient chairs, it's crucial to remain open to innovative advancements, ensuring you're not overly committed to a single brand.

TARGET COST
$4,000 - $8,000

(Opting for refurbished units can result in further savings.)

● OVER THE PATIENT (OTP) DELIVERY

A quick note on chair mounted delivery units, or Over the Patient (OTP) delivery as the ADA defines it. Chair mounted delivery, is probably the most common delivery method seen in practices today. Not surprisingly, and perhaps resulting from the fact, it also tends to be the most common (if not only) method of delivery used in dental Schools across the country. With a large predisposition towards its use it's not unsurprising that many dentists prefer this method of delivery especially established doctors who have been using it for several years. However, there are some noteworthy disadvantages to this particular delivery method that we should mention.

1) Utility cost. In order to use OTP delivery we need to run the dental utilities to the toe of the chair, compressed air at a minimum but sometimes dental water and vacuum as well. Since we often also have assistant utilities coming from the headwall (the suggested location for the assistant setup) this can add some redundancy to the room.

2) Equipment cost. Furthermore, the cost of a patient chair with a delivery arm is often $5k+ more than just a base chair. 3) Patient Experience. One of the most cited anxiety provoking experiences in the dental office for many patients is sitting in the chair and seeing the drills. Since we know the anxiety of patients directly correlates to their willingness to accept treatment, especially elective care, anything we can do to reduce this anxiety should have a beneficial impact on case acceptance. With that said, it's also worth mentioning that ergonomically, OTP delivery is actually fine as the worksurface often falls within the ideal Range of Motion outlined earlier. So if you have a strong preference towards using OTP, know that it shouldn't affect your physical performance too much but just be aware of some of the drawbacks it entails.

● WHERE SHOULD THE HANDPIECES GO?

9 out of 10 dental schools use over the patient handpieces with a pole mount light in their cubicles. Here's the reason why:

- They are easy to set up in a space that has no real walls.
- Performance doesn't matter to dental schools.
- Case presentation isn't a consideration.
- It's easy to swap the entire unit to a service area when it breaks.

● HERE IS THE TRUTH ABOUT OTP SETUPS

- They are absolutely OK 100%
- They are not the best for 4 handed treatment
- Apprehensive patients hate them.
- It's more difficult to do consultation in these rooms.
- Their use prevents the "Choose an ideal chair later" strategy

Over the patient handpieces are the average solution that will reliably produce adequate results. However, since you need a highly effective delivery & supply platform anyway, consider consolidating handpieces onto that platform.

Dental Light
LOW IMPACT

Some budding dentists might choose to sidestep dental lights initially. However, their significance in enhancing productivity deserves acknowledgment.

An independent light source, maneuverable by either the dentist or the assistant, proves invaluable. Imagine conducting a denture adjustment sans one! If you are hoping, like dental schools are, that dentures are going away and that everybody will be getting full mouth implants.. Think again! It's essential to cater to a diverse patient base, ensuring no segment feels overlooked.

Other factors to consider when deciding to use a dental light or not include loupes and headlamps. Generally speaking all providers (both doctors and hygienists) need adequate light sources in the oral cavity, so loupes can accommodate this for them, however assistants who find themselves working solo (polishing, bite checks, impressions, etc.) may find that they too need additional lighting. If we don't have dedicated dental lights then LED headlamps may be needed by these staff members. It's not uncommon for dentists to leave their rooms framed and wired to received dental lights in the future also, similar to the way some handle wall mounted X-rays.

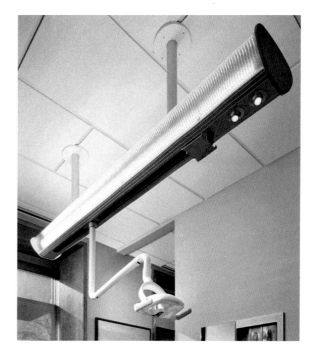

(Note: An operatory must have great general room lighting. While there exist innovative amalgamations of different light functionalities, these upgrades can be earmarked for future incorporation.) Install "blocking" to enable installments at a later date if you decide to omit at startup!

TARGET COST

$500 - $4,000

Assistant Sidewall
LOW IMPACT

This component primarily acts as a storage reservoir for supplemental items. This encompasses glove boxes, masks, headrest covers, and in-op sales products like electric toothbrushes, mouth rinses, whitening kits, etc. It may also furnish an auxiliary workspace in close proximity to the assistant. A cost-effective and functional approach to this would be adopting "lift-up" shelving, which saves a great deal of room width when compared to conventional fixed side cabinetry. If you plan appropriately in the design phase, these can be cut from the day 1 budget.

TARGET COST
$1,000 - $2,000

X-Ray
LOW IMPACT

The advent of handheld x-rays has marked a pivotal moment for emerging dental ventures. Thanks to significant advancements in battery technology, certain handheld x-rays now perform on par with their hard-wired counterparts, firing at 70kv, with the Carestream 4200p being a notable example as of this writing. One challenge is the need to charge these devices between shots, necessitating additional chargers for every operatory. Still, when you break down the costs, a single handheld x-ray can cater to three rooms, amounting to roughly $2,100 per room. In comparison, a wall-mounted x-ray would set you back by $3,500, indicating the economical advantage of handhelds. That being said, it's prudent to prepare for future upgrades; hence, ensuring the walls have the necessary support and power points for wall-mounted x-rays is advisable. This foresight will smoothen potential transitions, minimizing disruptions.

TARGET COST
$2,000 - $4,000

Nitrous Oxide
LOW IMPACT

For dental startups, mobility in nitrous oxide systems is a key factor to prioritize. Installing nitrous plumbing can be an expensive affair, potentially costing up to $5,000 per operatory, and this doesn't even factor in the flow meters. A more budget-friendly approach lies in opting for mobile setups, with several streamlined options available under $4,000.

The decision to go for nitrous oxide plumbing can be daunting, especially considering the soaring installation costs and the growing acceptance of oral sedatives. Many practitioners might find themselves contemplating its true necessity. However, from our vantage point, any dental practice intending to cater significantly to surgical, pediatrics, or apprehensive patients should view central nitrous oxide as indispensable.

TARGET COST
$4,000 - $50,000

THE REST OF THE OFFICE

Beyond the treatment rooms, which serve as the primary revenue generators, a range of support areas and systems play an equally crucial role in ensuring the smooth operation of a dental practice. As you delve deeper into the budget allocation for your office's overall infrastructure, these elements necessitate considerable attention. Striking a balance between your operatory expenses and these support systems might require revisiting some 'nice-to-have' features or even reconsidering the number of rooms you set up at the onset. A strategic approach would be to phase in rooms as your practice expands and cash flow becomes more robust. With the right planning during the design phase, adding equipment to pre-plumbed operatories in the future becomes a seamless transition, causing minimal disruption.

Compressor & Vacuum

Often referred to as the backbone of a dental practice, these systems are indispensable. A malfunction in a treatment room might cause a hiccup, but a breakdown in these foundational systems can bring your operations to a complete standstill. However, while they're vital, it doesn't necessarily mean you need the most expensive models. The emphasis should be on dependability. For air compressors, consider dual-headed units that offer redundancy, ensuring one can take over if the other fails. When it comes to efficiency, opting for a dry vacuum over a wet one is recommended, as it offers notable water savings.

Moreover, don't dismiss the potential value of high-quality, used, or refurbished units. Many practitioners, perhaps even including yourself, might find that their practices outgrow these mechanical systems well before they reach the end of their operational life. When sourced from credible vendors, these refurbished units can offer considerable savings without compromising on performance.

TARGET COST

$10,000 - $20,000.

Sterilization & Resupply

The sterilization area is the heart of your office. In this crucial space, you'll sterilize every instrument and keep all your operatories consistently stocked, ensuring they are always ready for procedures. The design of this room, grounded in a clear understanding of process and flow, is as vital as the equipment you choose to install.

For practices that utilize cassettes (which are highly effective, as detailed in our Blueprint to Maximizing Productivity), the sterilization process is straightforward. Your room design and equipment placement should mirror this linear approach. While many dealer reps and salespeople might advocate for "dental disinfector" washers, we believe they aren't worth their hefty price tag. Instead, we suggest commercial dishwashers. They are often half the cost of their dental equivalents, achieve higher water temperatures, and complete cycles in less time. Moreover, if a commercial dishwasher needs repairs, any local appliance technician can fix it, as opposed to specialized dental technicians. However, it's essential to consult your local regulatory body to ensure such appliances are permitted. (They are but your local authority might not believe so.)

On the other hand, investing in a quality autoclave upfront is wise. Choose a robust and reliable unit that can handle large batches at once. Opting for a sizable unit is beneficial because a smaller one will become a production bottleneck, increasing labor and reducing efficiency. Don't make this mistake!

Regarding the resupply component of this process, lower cabinets are generally unnecessary. Nearly half of your storage space is dedicated to bulk supplies, for which open shelving is more than adequate. Items like glove boxes, disinfectants, and headrest covers will occupy the majority of this space. Open tubs are excellent for organizing these products. For bulkier supplies, many practitioners prefer to store them in the original shipping boxes.

For smaller items, a more strategic approach is beneficial. We suggest adopting visual restocking techniques inspired by Lean manufacturing and the Toyota Production System. Transparent tilt bins are ideal for quickly gauging inventory levels, streamlining your monthly reorder process.

As a startup, optimizing every inch of your practice is pivotal. Why not utilize the often-overlooked vertical space in your resupply area? Hydraulic pull-down shelving can substantially augment your storage capacity. These units are not only practical but also safe and efficient. If budget constraints exist at the outset, these can be integrated later. Just ensure your initial design accommodates easy future installations through the planning of appropriate in wall blocking.

TARGET COST
$20,000 - $30,000

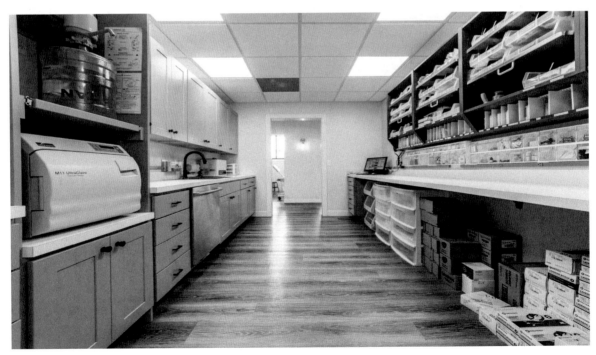

If you have the opportunity, move to an office-centric approach where inventory in centralized and everything is visual. You'll save time and money with this approach and it make resupply super easy using standardized checklists.

Lab

The requirements for a lab can differ significantly between practices. For instance, a pediatric office may only require a simple model trimmer positioned close to a sink. Contrastingly, a prosthodontist might desire a facility as comprehensive as the entire Glidewell research and development setup. For General Dentists embarking on a startup, we recommend establishing a compact, efficient analog lab. Importantly, this lab should be designed with a foresight for potential digital advancements. Presently, a fully digital lab may entail some costly investments and is not something that a startup with limited funds should underwrite.

At its core, this modest analog lab should include a model trimmer, vacuum former, glazing oven, lathe, workbench/area with handpieces, and a dust collection system. Ensure that space is available for a potential milling unit and glazing oven. Also, ample space for both incoming and outgoing case pans, which hold impressions and study models, is vital. The intricacies in design are critical to achieve efficiency. Collaborate closely with your office designer to ensure your specific needs are addressed.

TARGET COST

$5,000 - $50,000

Digital Imaging, CAD/CAM

When considering Panoramic and, potentially, 3D CBCT units, upgradeability should be the primary concern for startups. A few imaging brands, notably Carestream, have innovated products that can be upgraded throughout their life cycle. For instance, you can begin with a basic 2D pan for approximately $25,000. If later you decide to delve into advanced diagnostics and implants, the same unit can be upgraded to a 3D model for an added $40,000. Even though this method might be $15,000 pricier than initially purchasing the most affordable 3D model, it's a strategy that can prove economical over 2-3 years. During this period, you can amass a patient base, hone your clinical prowess, and offset your practice debt.

TARGET COST

$25,000 - $100,000

SUMMARY

There are numerous other products and equipment pieces to consider. However, we aimed to delve into these pivotal ones. A thorough New Office Purchasing Checklist, complete with recommended items and their prices, can be found in the Resources section. This list is adaptable to individual needs and serves as a budgeting guide.

11 SUPPLIES & INVENTORY

After securing major equipment, the subsequent significant expenditure is the initial inventory purchase. This initial stock will equip your office with operative supplies, consumables, and administrative inventory for an estimated 4-6 weeks.

A 4-6 week inventory target is ideal as it facilitates a large monthly order for primary items. This cycle not only aids in budgeting but also serves as an indicator of your consumption rate for particular supplies. For instance, if you consistently deplete stock of a certain item before the month's end, this pattern highlights a need to reassess and possibly increase the Minimum Stock Level (MSL) for that item. Conversely, if you consistently end the month with excess of another item, it may be prudent to decrease its MSL.

A well-maintained inventory spreadsheet is an invaluable tool to track and manage stock levels. Key components of an inventory spreadsheet include:

- **Item #**

- **Unit:** Size or volume of the product.

- **Description:** Brief description of the item.

- **Vendor:** Supplier or source of the item.

- **Price:** Cost per unit size.

- **MSL (Minimum Stock Level):** The lowest quantity of a product that must be on hand.

- **QOH (Quantity on Hand):** Current stock level of the item.

- **Order Amt:** Quantity to order, calculated by subtracting QoH from MSL.

- **Total:** Total cost of items to order, derived from Order Amt multiplied by Price.

- **Location 1:** Primary location for immediate use (e.g., tub, bin).

- **Location 2:** Backup or storage location (e.g., sterilization area, cabinet).

Your physical organization of supplies should mirror the spreadsheet's structure. By categorizing items based on their use, you can efficiently navigate both the storage area and the spreadsheet in a systematic manner. Most materials and supplies should be visually accessible, a concept we elaborate on in our Guide to Maximizing Productivity. This visibility facilitates a quick visual inventory assessment against the spreadsheet. By incorporating a basic IF formula in Excel, items that dip below the MSL are automatically flagged with their order amount in the spreadsheet. Conversely, items at or above the MSL will not prompt an order amount, leaving their respective fields blank. This system ensures efficient restocking and reduces the potential for supply shortages or overstocking.

When starting, your Quantity on Hand (QOH) for every item will be zero. In our sample inventory list, we've provided placeholder values for the Minimum Stock Level suitable for a 6-operatory practice. It's essential to scrutinize this list, removing items you don't use and updating vendor details and pricing as needed. Still, it offers a helpful baseline to begin.

Though it may be tempting to explore various vendors for the best prices, consolidating your purchases can simplify operations immensely. Historically, after comparing two or three major suppliers every year, we've found that Darby Dental consistently offers better rates than Patterson & Schein. When handling an inventory list of 250-500 items, reducing the number of vendors streamlines the purchasing, receiving, stocking, and deployment processes. Furthermore, for new employees, understanding the inventory becomes easier when there's consistency in the products used and their sources. Considering that supplies usually constitute 5%-8% of the entire office budget, spending excessive hours each month to save a marginal 1% doesn't justify the effort.

However, it's important to emphasize that we do not recommend bulk buying as a cost-saving strategy. The space consumed by bulk items can negate any potential financial benefits, as this area could be more productively utilized. It might seem appealing to purchase a pallet of glove boxes at a discount, but the minute you need that storage space for another purpose, like setting up an additional treatment room, you'll find yourself relocating that pallet, perhaps even to your personal garage. A six-week supply is generally all that's necessary. It ensures that you don't over-purchase, reduces the risk of products expiring, and makes it easier to swap out or eliminate obsolete or redundant items.

For a comprehensive list of startup supplies, please refer to our "Start-Up Supply" section in the Resources.

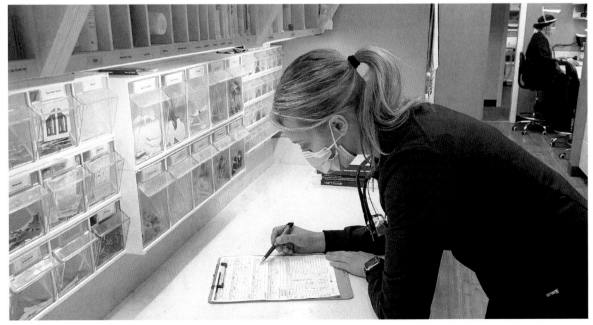

If you have the opportunity, move to an office-centric approach where inventory in centralized and everything is visual. You'll save time and money with this approach and it make resupply super easy using standardized checklists.

12 HIRING, TRAINING & RETENTION

Starting your dental practice and hiring your first team can be daunting. Here's a simple roadmap to guide you through the process.

1. **Administrators**

   Start with an administrator. This person will be instrumental in setting up foundational systems and handling the paperwork that becomes necessary as the team grows. Their primary responsibilities will include:
   - Setting up payroll services.
   - Posting job advertisements, filtering resumes, and assisting with interviews.
   - Onboarding and training new employees on the practice management software.
   - Answering phone calls.

2. **Dental Assistants** (You'll need two)

   Once the administrative foundation is set, you'll need dental assistants. Their responsibilities encompass:
   - Managing and ordering dental inventory.
   - Familiarizing themselves with your case presentation style and preferences.
   - Handling new patient intake, managing health history forms, x-rays, and taking impressions.
   - Assisting with all dental procedures.

3. **Dental Hygienists** (Aim for two)

   Hygienists play a crucial role in the patient experience. Their tasks include:
   - Being the primary point of contact for new patient visits.
   - Completing new patient checklists and exam slips.
   - Conducting routine cleanings (prophies) and periodontal treatments daily.
   - Administering local anesthesia (L.A.) if the doctor is unavailable.

This basic structure is the heart of any dental practice. While specific details might change, this foundational layout remains consistent whether your practice is just starting or has been running for a decade.

As your practice grows and patient volume increases, you'll inevitably need to expand your team. For insights on how to manage and anticipate this growth, check out our video on "Math of Staff Growth." This resource illustrates the evolution of a budding practice into a thriving, established one. Once you reach this 'Golden Age,' your goals will determine the trajectory of your practice.

To better understand the dynamics of growth, consider the "Math of Growth." This conceptual framework explains how a surge in new patients eventually results in a majority of regular, recall patients. Practices that have been operating for 5-10 years might recognize this scenario: a packed hygiene schedule dominated by recall appointments, which can reduce opportunities for new patient intake. This shift can sometimes depress both hygiene and doctor production due to fewer comprehensive exams and significant dental treatments.

Our "Math of Staff Growth" spreadsheet provides a clear overview of the staffing needs at various stages of practice growth. While your immediate focus might be on the early growth stages (expanding from 5 to 7 chairs and then from 7 to 10), it's beneficial to have a long-term perspective. Remember, today's large corporations began as smaller entities.

The **Math** of **Growth**

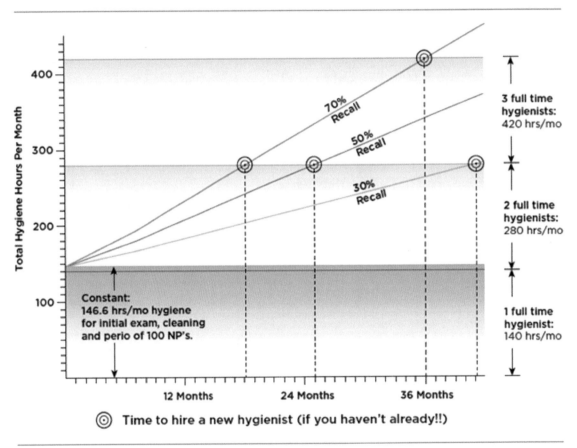

It can be easy as a start-up practice to lose sight of the need to accommodate future growth.

"Heart Charts" are a tool we've designed, drawing inspiration from the Kanban concept of visual inspection. We've tailored it to suit employee training and evaluation. Every role—whether it's an assistant, front desk representative, or hygienist—has a progression ladder to climb. From the day of hiring until achieving "Master" level status, there's always a new skill to acquire, an area to improve, or additional value to bring to the practice. This chart succinctly maps out these progression steps, allowing a clear view of each employee's current position. It serves dual purposes: it applauds achievements and promotions, and it identifies areas where coaching or even reprimands might be needed. For instance, if two assistants are hired simultaneously, and after three months one has achieved 7 hearts while the other only 3, it provides a clear, transparent basis for discussing their performance. Often, employees will self-assess in light of these metrics—either eagerly striving for the next milestone or opting to pursue opportunities elsewhere.

Another pivotal tool in our toolkit, especially when assessing job candidates, is the "Right Fit" profile concept by Kathy Kolbe. In essence, the Right Fit profile posits that individuals inherently excel in certain roles more than others, and these inclinations can be gauged, particularly through personality tests. In early 2015, we conducted these tests on staff across several of our top-performing dental practices.

The findings, elaborated in Dr. David Ahearn's lecture "Who Are All These People?", were remarkable. In virtually every practice and in virtually every role, distinct personality types clustered together. While we had anticipated some patterns, the extensive correlations across diverse organizations, located in different states with entirely unique teams, were beyond our expectations.

With this invaluable insight, we crafted a tailored Right Fit Profile™ for each role within our organization. During interviews, especially when weighing the merits of multiple competent candidates, we can juxtapose them against this standard profile. Experience has shown that 95% of the time, aligning with this profile indicates a much greater chance for a successful fit for the designated position.

However, it's essential to clarify: this isn't the foremost deciding element in our hiring process. And, it's critical to approach with caution, as some jurisdictions are skeptical about the use of such tests in employment decisions. While the Right Fit Profile is undeniably a potent tool for forecasting future performance, our selection criteria takes into account other aspects as well. Candidates are primarily assessed on their experience, inherent personality, professional demeanor, references, and other unique factors like philanthropic activities or significant accomplishments. Remember, we are all "Caregivers."

Even with these systems in place, some turnover is an inevitable part of the business. People move, leave to raise families, etc. Nevertheless, these mechanisms transform the hiring paradigm. Instead of it being an unpredictable gamble, it evolves into a more methodical approach, seeking to consistently produce optimal outcomes.

13 MARKETING & BRANDING

When launching a startup marketing campaign, there are two pivotal activities: Planning and Running a Campaign, and Measuring the Results. It's crucial to establish a marketing budget and adhere to it. The CWA 2021 report states that the average marketing budget for a GP practice is 1.75% of revenue. This percentage is averaged over all GP practices in their database, many of which are likely established. A brand-new startup should increase this percentage until a patient base forms and the percentage of monthly patient referrals begins to grow. For a startup, we recommend allocating 3% of your budget to marketing, which would equate to $2,500/mo assuming annual revenue of $1M.

NAME & LOGO

Choosing a name for your first practice can be daunting. Most experts advise a straightforward approach, suggesting names that clearly state what you offer. While names like "Divine Dentistry" might sound appealing due to their alliteration, they might give potential patients the wrong impression unless you are genuinely offering boutique or spa-like services. Names such as "Destination Dental" and "Darn Good Dentistry" might also mislead. Instead, consider names that resonate with the location of your practice. Titles like "Southcoast Smiles," "Blue Ridge Dental," or "Lakeview Dental" can help anchor your practice in the minds of your patients.

While many dental practices are named after their owners, like "Smith Dental Associates" or "Ahearn Dental Care", this might present challenges in the future. If you transition to an associate-driven practice and you're not actively seeing patients, clients might be hesitant to visit. This potential issue can be sidestepped by opting for a more neutral office name. (As a side note, Dr. Ahearn never named his practice "Ahearn Dental" because he knew that people couldn't figure out how to pronounce his name!)

Always check your desired business name against existing registrations in your state to ensure it's available. Other dentists will notice your marketing efforts, and if they view your name as too similar to theirs, they could take legal action, which might force a name change on your part. It's a risk worth avoiding.

For your logo, engage a graphic artist to produce 4-6 design concepts once you've decided on a name. Share these designs with a diverse group to gauge reactions and gather feedback. Aim for a logo that resonates with your target demographic, like mothers, spouses, and professionals. It should also be simple and easily replicable in print—avoid designs that are overly intricate or large.

WEBSITE

Your website will be the primary touchpoint for most prospective patients—it's the cornerstone of your marketing communication. Almost every potential new patient will search for you online before making that first call. Hence, it's vital to present a website that's professional, user-friendly, and informative, focusing on the following essential elements:

1. **Your phone number**
   Make it prominent and clickable to facilitate ease of communication.

2. **A welcome video**
   This could be a personalized introduction by you or a staff member, or perhaps a voice-over accompanying a visual tour or dynamic images.

3. **An enticing offer**
   Startups should seriously consider using a discounted promotion! Include a clear call-to-action. Classic offers such as "Free Exam & X-rays with Insurance" have a proven track record of success. Other effective promotions might include "Cleanings from $X", "Whitening from $X", or "No Insurance? No Worries! Check Out Our Patient Care Program". For tailored marketing strategies, specialized companies like Chris Ad can be consulted.

4. **Essential information**
   Display your core details such as operational hours, team introductions, an office tour (if aesthetically appealing), and the services you provide. Research local competitors' websites and note the features you admire and those you'd prefer to avoid. Share this feedback with your website developer.

Critical Point: If you're partnering with a website design firm, ensure that YOU retain ownership of the content and its associated rights, indefinitely.

Regarding online appointment booking, while this feature is appreciated by many, we're yet to be completely convinced that is the right way to schedule a startup. That is the right way to schedule a startup. Our reservations stem from concerns about potential no-shows and the sight of an empty calendar.

SOCIAL MEDIA

It's impossible to discuss modern marketing without addressing the behemoth that is social media. When executed effectively, social media platforms can broadcast your content and brand message to tens of thousands daily. However, a poorly-managed presence can deter potential patients.

Given the ever-changing nature of these platforms, precise advice is a challenge. But at the very least, having active profiles on Facebook, Instagram, and perhaps LinkedIn is advisable. Some practices also thrive on platforms like TikTok and Snapchat, but these demand a more intensive content creation approach.

Consider YouTube if you're inclined to produce regular, engaging 'infotainment' (informational and entertaining) content. Not only does this provide value to viewers, but it also bolsters your website's SEO ranking.

Our recommendation: designate a dedicated team member to oversee social media endeavors... But choose carefully! Even if it's a part-time role initially, regular check-ins and monthly strategy sessions are crucial. Ensure you're involved in the content creation process and request monthly updates on performance metrics and insights. This hands-on approach will be vital when evaluating the success of your marketing strategies in the 'Measuring Your

Results' segment. Do realize however that "free" social media marketing" - is actually quite expensive to do it well - because of the labor involved.

DIRECT MAIL

From our extensive experience with dental office startups, expansions, and new constructions, direct mail emerges as a powerful yet intricate tool. As one of the pricier marketing avenues on this list, it also often turns out to be the predominant source of new patients for practices that invest in it. In some cases, it attracts 2 to 3 times as many new patients as any other singular approach.

With a marketing budget set at $2,500 per month, aiming for 40 new patients means roughly $62 per new patient. A typical direct mail campaign might demand $200-$300 for every new patient acquired. Our advice: initially invest in a batch of 10,000 mailers (about $4,000) and then hit the pause button until the practice's cash flow can accommodate further investment.

Let's run the numbers: at $200-$300 per patient with a 3% marketing budget, you'd require these new patients to represent over $5,000 in treatments to stay within budget constraints. For a startup, this expectation may be lofty. But remember, each new patient's acquisition cost is impacted by your referral rate. With a 50% referral percentage (meaning for every 2 new patients, one comes from a referral), your real cost plummets. Taking the $200 new patient cost and multiplying it by a 50% referral rate gives you an actual cost of $100 per patient. With your 3% marketing budget, this translates to a more realistic $3,300 average case value. It's still ambitious, but much more attainable.

PATIENT GIFTS

One subtle yet impactful recommendation we consistently make is gifting each new patient.

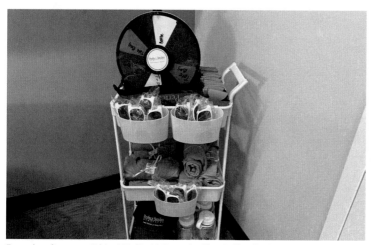

Drawing from Cialdini's 6 Rules of Influence, the principle of Reciprocity stands out. Offering a gift, no matter how modest, instills a sense of indebtedness in the patient. This emotional trigger can lead to greater case acceptances, increased referral rates, or even more candid feedback.

There's no need for extravagant gestures. Given a $62 budget per new patient, a give-away worth about $20 strikes the right balance. The ideal gift is something that won't end up in

Examples of swag available at Dr. David Ahearn's office, Perfect Smiles Dentistry.

the trash and will see frequent use: beach towels, fleece blankets, stuffed toys, travel mugs, refrigerator magnets, USB thumb drives, or travel care cases. Items that become part of daily routines, especially those bearing your logo, are ideal. They not only serve as a constant reminder of your practice but also often become inadvertent marketing tools in their own right.

Other people will see this and may prompt conversation and questions.

B2B OUTREACH

In the early days of your startup, one worthwhile strategy involves engaging with local businesses in your vicinity. Consider putting together a gift basket filled with oral care essentials such as toothbrushes, toothpaste, floss, mouth rinse, and a patient gift. Topping it off with a $50 off treatment card can be a nifty addition. Before making your visit, ring up these businesses to inquire about their number of employees. Your sweet spot would be companies that boast 30-50 employees, ideally with dental insurance provisions.

When delivering your curated basket, ensure it lands in the hands of influential personnel— preferably the director of HR or a senior manager. A front desk representative might not have the clout to make decisions or disseminate the information effectively. Take the opportunity to ask if they already have a designated dental provider. If the answer is no, express your interest in becoming their preferred choice. If you're broaching this topic, it's crucial to ascertain beforehand that you accept their insurance, aligning with the principle of Reciprocity.

TV & RADIO

Venture into television and radio advertising after you've exhausted or established the previously mentioned marketing strategies. Historically, they're more challenging to measure in terms of ROI but can be incredibly effective in the right circumstances.

Both TV and radio have a knack for resonating with specific demographic segments. In almost every locale, there's that one news channel that families tune into each evening, or a radio station that commuters religiously listen to during their drives. Your task is to identify these platforms, zero in on the most impactful time slots, and understand the cost structure for 30-second advertisements. Many stations offer packages bundling multiple ad spots spread across weeks or even months. Some might even feature web-based segments or those anchored by prominent personalities. Engaging in longer commitments often fetches additional discounts.

An essential metric to track is the viewership or listenership in your targeted area or zip code. Given the broad outreach of these mediums, anticipate a conversion rate lower than 1% and evaluate the ROI based on that. While TV and radio might command higher new patient acquisition costs compared to Direct Mail, they can yield exceptional results if you're the sole dentist advertising on a renowned channel or station.

MEASURING THE RESULTS

Having outlined our marketing campaign and set a budget, it's essential that we measure the results of our efforts. While this isn't an exact science – given that potential new patients might have come across our marketing materials in multiple locations before deciding to seek our services – it's still crucial to determine the most effective strategies. Their "referral source" might merely be the last one they recall when completing their new patient form.

Nevertheless, we must allocate our budget and identify which marketing activities have the greatest impact. One efficient way to gather this information is through the New Patient Intake form. While this data can also be collected during the initial phone call, the form serves as a backup in case the phone team misses this detail.

To avoid overwhelming the patients with too many choices, we typically provide the following options on the form:

HOW DID YOU HEAR ABOUT US?

☐ Friend / Family / Colleague
Who can we thank for the referral? _____

☐ Office Sign / Walk In

☐ Direct Mail

☐ Internet / Web Search

☐ Social Media

☐ TV / Radio

☐ Other _____

We label the "Referral Source" for every new patient within our practice management software and generate a monthly report, summarizing the data. This information is then transferred to a straightforward spreadsheet, from which we plot graphs.

This allows us to quickly discern which marketing efforts are improving, declining, or remaining consistent. We recommend augmenting the spreadsheet with additional metrics such as total new patients (NPs), overall production, and the expense for each category. This facilitates calculations for NP acquisition cost and production per referral source. By dividing the production by the expense, we can compute the Return on Investment (ROI).

It's also worth noting that our calculations incorporate our Referral Percentage rate. Thus, the value of each new patient is essentially 1 plus our referral percentage.

14 GRAND OPENING

PHOTOSHOOT

As we prepare for our Grand Opening Day and its subsequent announcement, we must ensure we have professional photographs of the office. Based on our experience in setting up offices, we understand that the office looks its best on Day 0. Therefore, we shouldn't miss this prime opportunity to capture its essence.

Hiring a professional photographer is crucial. They will expertly stage the rooms, fine-tune the lighting, apply appropriate filters, and craft images that exude a "Wow" factor. These photographs will not only serve your marketing needs but will also grace our social media platforms and populate the "Office Tour" section of our website. A key suggestion: incorporate smiling individuals in your photos to convey warmth and approachability. Note: We provide this service complimentary to our design & equipment clients.

SOFT OPENING

We highly recommend hosting a "soft opening" on the Thursday or Friday preceding your official Grand Opening, slated for the subsequent week. This soft opening, essentially offering complimentary cleanings to friends and family, provides an invaluable chance to iron out any operational wrinkles under a full schedule. It prompts several questions: Is the software functioning optimally? Can hygiene exams be completed promptly? How effective were the diagnoses and their presentations? Were the assistants adept in handling equipment and preparing rooms efficiently? Above all, did the system run seamlessly?

It's imprudent to "go live" without this preliminary test run. If there are glitches to uncover, it's far better to identify them with a familiar and understanding crowd, rather than with a genuine patient needing extensive dental care worth over $5k.

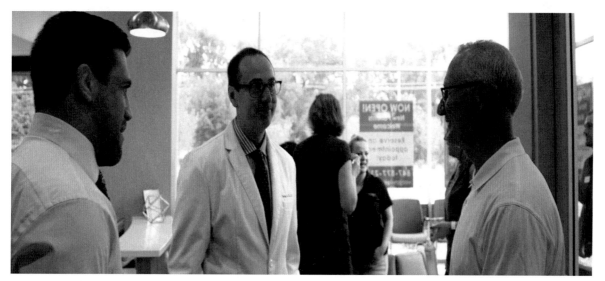

T Dr. Peter Kics of Westgate Dental Care greets friends, family, and members of the community at an Open House event. The team at Tend Dental made their Open House event an opportunity to create a presence in their community.

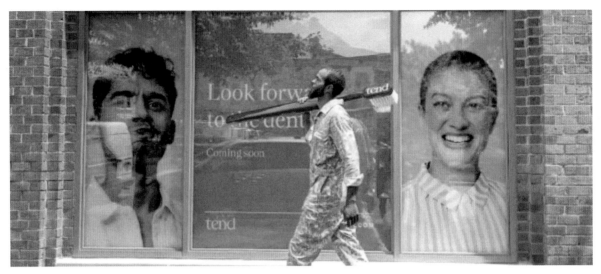

The team at Tend Dental made their Open House event an opportunity to create a presence in their community.

GRAND OPENING

Assuming the soft opening unfolds smoothly, and our marketing campaign has yielded some advance appointments, we're set for the real deal: the Grand Opening. The schedule for this day should be relatively relaxed, perhaps seeing 1 or 2 patients hourly for exams, x-rays, treatment planning, and case presentations. A noteworthy tip: Reaching out to local officials, such as the mayor or state representatives, might result in them attending for a ribbon-cutting ceremony. This gesture could garner media attention and offer invaluable free publicity for the new office's inauguration.

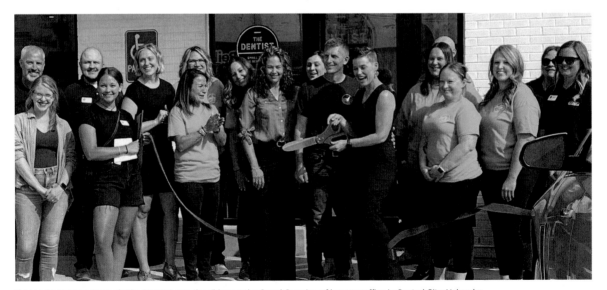

Kristen Hermansen-Ryan of "The Dentist" cuts the ribbon at the Grand Opening of her new office in Central City, Nebraska.

CHECKLIST

- [ ] 1. Financial Health Check
- [ ] 2. Create Business Plan
- [ ] 3. Obtain Financing
- [ ] 4. Find Location
- [ ] 5. Negotiate Lease
- [ ] 6. Develop Test Fit Diagram
- [ ] 7. Develop Floor Plan
- [ ] 8. Developer Interior Design
- [ ] 9. Choose Dental Equipment
- [ ] 10. Develop MEP's/Permit Plans
- [ ] 11. Hire Contractor/Pull Permits
- [ ] 12. Start Construction
- [ ] 13. Install Dental Equipment
- [ ] 14. Test & Train
- [ ] 15. Soft Opening
- [ ] 16. Grand Opening

15 ADDITIONAL RESOURCES

Sample P&L's by Cain Watters & Associates

Sample Business Plan by Design Ergonomics

Sample Cash Flow Projections by Tim Gagnon

Sample Letter of Intent by Design Ergonomics

18 Elements of an Ideal General Practice Floor Plan by Design Ergonomics

Sample Floor Plan by Design Ergonomics

New Office Purchasing Checklist by Design Ergonomics

Start-Up Supply Checklist by Design Ergonomics

Your Blueprint for Maximizing Dental Office Productivity by Dr. David Ahearn

Construction Calculator by Tim Gagnon

Math of Growth by Tim Gagnon

Math of Staff Growth by Tim Gagnon

Heart Chart Template by Design Ergonomics

These helpful resources are available for downloading, free of charge, at:

https://desergo.com/start-up-materials

or by scanning the QR code below.

Made in the USA
Las Vegas, NV
05 November 2024

11198956R00050